STAR MEDICINE

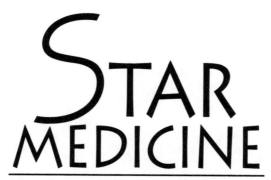

STAR MEDICINE

Native American Path to Emotional Healing

WOLF MOONDANCE
Illustrated by Jim Sharpe & Sky Starhawk

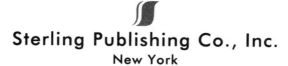

Sterling Publishing Co., Inc.
New York

By the same author
RAINBOW MEDICINE
SPIRIT MEDICINE

Library of Congress Cataloging-in-Publication Data
Moondance, Wolf.
    Star medicine : Native American path to emotional healing / Wolf
Moondance ; illustrated by Jim Sharpe & Sky Starhawk.
       p.   cm.
    Includes index.
    ISBN 0-8069-9547-5
    1. Shamanism—United States—Miscellanea.   2. Medicine wheels—
Miscellanea.   3. Spiritual life.   I. Title.
BF1622.U6M67   1997
299'.7—dc21   97-1003
                                                 CIP

10 9 8 7 6 5 4

Published by Sterling Publishing Company, Inc.
387 Park Avenue South, New York, N.Y. 10016
© 1997 by Wolf Moondance
Additional illustrations © 1997 by Jim Sharpe
Distributed in Canada by Sterling Publishing
% Canadian Manda Group, One Atlantic Avenue, Suite 105
Toronto, Ontario, Canada M6K 3E7
Distributed in Great Britain and Europe by Cassell PLC
Wellington House, 125 Strand, London WC2R 0BB, England
Distributed in Australia by Capricorn Link (Australia) Pty Ltd.
P.O. Box 6651, Baulkham Hills, Business Centre, NSW 2153, Australia
Manufactured in the United States of America
All rights reserved

Sterling ISBN 0-8069-9547-5

Dedication

With heartfelt gratitude, a freedom in my heart, I dedicate this book to
Joe Cake, XO.

Contents

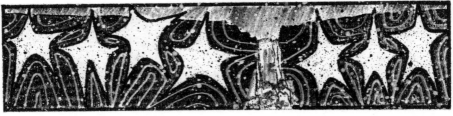

Success Medicine Teaching
Coup Stick
The Process of the Lesson of Poise

The Emotional Teachings of Happy
Ceremony of the Yellow Bird —
    Building a Vision Square
Spirit Shirt Vision of the Hawk
Vision Medicine
The Process of the Lesson
    of Discipline

The Emotional Teachings of Sad
Ceremony of the Evergreen
Spirit Shirt Vision of the Dragonfly
Herb Bundles
Beauty Medicine Teaching
The Process of the Lesson of Account

The Emotional Teachings of Anger
Ceremony of the Moon—A Healing Circle
Super Shirt Vision of the Frog
Medicine Rocks
The Process of the Lesson of Fact
Healing Medicine

The Emotional Teachings of Fear
Ceremony of the Stars —
    Wishing on a Star
Spirit Shirt Vision of the Owl
Spirit Pouch of Power
Ceremony of the Silver Star Pouch
Using a Star
The Process of the Lesson of Sense of Self
Power Medicine

Purpose

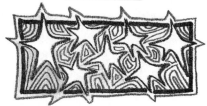

Star Medicine is the third book in the series of *Rainbow Medicine*. It is the second section of the medicine wheel, known as the South. It is the emotions. It is the color green. It is the summertime. It is the dance of the Rainbow Self. Standing in the gateway of the South, you are overseen by the spirit guide of the coyote. It was given to me a long time ago when I was a child—a vision of the sun, the moon, and the seven stars. I walked with that vision and came to a place where I saw a medicine wheel being remembered. It was a vision given to a wise grandfather who saw people and animals coming together in a circle. Many times in my life I have come across different teachings of medicine wheels. There are many beliefs that people live with. It is mine that, as the seven stars spoke to me, they brought forth seven sacred teachings. I call them medicines and they hold hands with lessons. For it is a lesson in life that we have the medicine to treat, and it is a medicine that we understand and can treat those lessons with our faith.

There is much controversy in our lives and it is because of emotions. We all have our feelings, we all have our teachings. We all have been taught different things through the years of our lives. No matter how young or old we are, we have opinions, and opinions are made up of feelings, and feelings are emotions. When we stand in the south gate we are facing our emotions, and within the south part of the Rainbow Medicine Wheel we can understand the depth of our emotions. The Rainbow Medicine Wheel itself is based on four directions of sevens and seven sets of teachings. This is the second set.

First there is Spirit medicine, and that is the East. This, the second, is Star Medicine; it is about the emotions and that is the South. It is my purpose to bring you the understanding of such tools as a spirit journal and prayer ties, and a ceremony of the herbs known as smudging. It is my purpose to give you an understanding of some of the spirit guides and connections of the South, an understanding of honoring the South, and the seven stars in the South that are medicines. One is known as the Dance of the Red Rose, which is Strength medicine; it has with it the lesson of Clarity. The second stone, the orange stone, is the Dance of the Earth,

Success medicine, and with it is the process of the lesson of Poise. The third is the Dance of the Yellow Bird, which is Vision medicine and has with it the process of the lesson of Discipline. The fourth is the Dance of the Evergreen, which is Beauty medicine and has with it the process of the lesson of Account. The fifth is the Dance of the Moon, Healing medicine, and with it the process of the lesson of Fact. The sixth is the Dance of the Stars. It is Power medicine and with it is the process of the lesson of Sense. The seventh is the Dance of the Great Waterfall, Great medicine with the process of the lesson of Complete.

Standing in the south gate, looking towards the north, there is a straight line of color—red, orange, yellow, green, blue, purple, and burgundy. It is laid down, one rock at a time, for the lessons—the lesson of Clarity, of Poise, of Discipline, of Account, of Fact, of Sense, and of Complete. Moving clockwise in the medicine wheel, we step on each star, which is a stone, and there are seven of them—Strength, Success, Vision, Beauty, Healing, Power, and Great.

In bringing forth the depth of my vision of the sun, the moon, and the seven stars, I bring a contemporary way, an alternative healing, a shamanic movement through spiritual guidance that allows us to transform our emotions.

Transforming our emotions is a dance of spirit. Among Native American people, dancing is a very important process of life. It is both physical and spiritual. Dance is the discipline of prayer in a physical form. It is our Sense and our Complete. It is a way of life that brings happiness into our hearts and souls, that allows our spirit to maintain its walk on this earth as a two-legged. I say "contemporary" because it is now.

I make no claim that this book is traditional medicine of any breed or race of Native American heritage. No teachers sat me down and taught me these ways. They came to me through the voices of the stars and they are my teaching as a shaman. Shamanism is my belief, and I have walked as a shaman for many years. As you read these words, you may recognize things someone else has already told you. That's because Rainbow Medicine is a rainbow. It comes from Great Spirit as a promise that we will never be destroyed, but will always be uplifted in light.

Emotions are what the south part of the wheel is about. And the purpose of Star Medicine is for us to reach within the stars and hold on to the point. And the point of this book is that we put away our racism, that we lay down our anger. We do that through Confidence and Balance, through Creativity, through Growth, through Truth, through Wisdom, and through Impeccability. Our emotions—whether we're black, yellow, red, or white—are our driving force. It is my purpose through these chapters to help you to move within the Rose and walk upon the Earth; to fly with the Yellow Bird; to stand solid with the Evergreen; to rise with the Moon; to walk on the Stars; to flow with the Waterfall. For to me, these are my family.

It is in the Dance of the Rainbow Self, through this contemporary movement, that I have spent my life and dedicated my heart, my walk, and my emotions. It is the way that I bring honor to elders—aunties and uncles, grandmothers, and grandfathers—and it is the way that each of you will find a song within your heart as you walk within Star Medicine. Then you will have found a Native American path to bring about a healing of your emotions. You may have tears, and they may be of joy or happiness; they may be of sadness and grief; they may be of anger and bitterness, but you will take them and dance them, knowing that they will bring you closer to Great Spirit.

Within the Rainbow Medicine Wheel we have the four directions of life. When you have understood the four directions, you have stood with two males and two females, you have walked in the balance of a double Yin/Yang. So it is not just of this country that this book speaks; it is not of this earth that this book speaks, for it is beyond there—beyond the Milky Way. Across the Rainbow Bridge. For emotions come from feelings and feelings come from thoughts, and thoughts are the breath of God, Great Spirit, Grandmother, Grandfather, Holy Spirit, Creator.

It is my knowing that, as the water moves over the Great Falls, each drop is a brother/sister as each one of us is a point of light. Within these teachings of the emotions, I wish for us all to feel as we read. To feel the open doors of red, orange, yellow, green, blue, purple, and burgundy. To feel Star Medicine guiding, transforming, bringing forth within the growth and healing of the existence of every one of us.

Aho.

Prelude

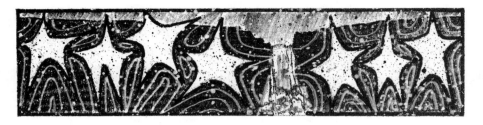

Around a small fire dances one with tears in her eyes, one who is alone, one whose feet press down on the Earth Mother, one after another. She sings a song with Grandmother spirit in her heart as the wind circles around and around—a song of one who grows stronger. There is lightning and thunder, wind, and rain. The fire burns. And the one dances.

The dance is known as life and the one that dances is a hollow bone, a human two-legged who is open to all worlds and the will of Great Spirit. Every one of us is given the opportunity to live the fullness of our existence as a two-legged. The mystery school of life is known as the wheel, the sacred circle, the sacred hoop. We are called to that by goodness. We are called to existence by life. And that one who dances and sings, steps through the south gate, passing in and out through spirit and the physical. Standing in her present form, she is one who walks the medicine road and feels. Emotions are those feelings. They allow one to be. Oh, yeah, she carries the carcass with her; she has the bones and the blood and the muscle. They are feelings. They are emotions.

Within Star Medicine, the Dance of the Rainbow Self is brought forth as a knowing. What is it all about? What does it matter? Maybe I will and maybe I won't. What if I do and what if I don't? Ah, there is more to life than that. There is more to life than maybe I will and maybe I won't. But if your emotions are weakened, and there is a lack of strength, then it will be "maybe." And if you have a fear of success, then it will be weakness and it will be "What if I do and what if I don't?" It's up to you. It's up to you to decide if you're going to give up and lie down in life or if you're going to stand up and dance.

It's up to you. The wind whistles around your head, the stars call your name. The stars *are* your name. Your medicine is not what if you do or what if you don't. Your medicine is the Dance of the Rainbow Self. The honor of the south gate—looking the coyote in the face, knowing your innocence, and holding on to it. It is understanding Acceptance and being in Acceptance, and feeling Disgust and accepting Disgust. It allows you to bring about your Poise, where you stand in the lesson of Clarity, and open yourself. There, Happiness and Joy are your Ceremony of the Yellow Bird.

The sweet smell of the Evergreen—the pine scents whisper through your mind. Sad it's not. It is life, fullness. Beauty. Anger may rip and tear and stop the dance. Rain can put out the fire, but it is healing medicine, the Dance of the Moon, that gives you the lesson of Fact and you can analyze and judge for yourself. You have the lesson of Account.

In emotions, anger is real. It is a process in which you may turn in disgust and say, "Yuck!" But it is a place where you don't have to stay with your head dropped down and your pride broken. Anger will motivate you, unless you break, unless you quit, unless you give up. Unless you allow fear to endure. The Dance of the Stars gives you Power medicine—the medicine to look the owl in the face and not be afraid of death—to stand up to the prophecies and understand tomorrow. There are the lessons of Sense. Does it make sense to stick your hand in the fire? That's your choice of liquor and drugs. Emotions of fear sometimes save your life and allow you to dance the Dance of the Great Waterfall—that gives you the emotions of Great medicine, of Joy—the greatest medicine of all. It allows you the lesson of Complete.

You sit with the seven lessons of the self when you look at the primary emotions. The lesson of Acceptance lies before you. The lesson of Disgust, the lesson of Happy, the lesson of Sad, the lesson of Anger, the lesson of Fear, and the lesson of Joy—all lie before you.

Into the Medicine Wheel

There are many medicine wheels throughout the teachings of Native philosophy. There are medicine wheels that not even traditional Native Americans know the teachings of. Medicine wheel teachings are known as the Mystery School, and the Mystery School extends into all beliefs. Every belief has its mysteries. Within the medicine wheel mysteries become known. They become the Great; they become Impeccable; they become Grand; they become the Will of Great Spirit. Many things in life want to be known—the powers, the forces, the callings. It is in the medicine wheel that you can bring things to life in a spiritual way.

A medicine wheel is a place where you step inside of All. When you stand in the center, you are standing in All. A medicine wheel starts with a point and resonates in a clockwise, circular motion, opening up gateways.

This is how your energy moves through your life, from your spirit, your emotions, your body, and your mind.

Within the medicine wheel are the four parts of the self. Where the wheel represents the circle, the circle represents the total self. When working with the Rainbow Medicine Wheel, always enter it through the East and acknowledge your spirit.

As you walk in the medicine wheel you always move clockwise, for positive energy travels in a clockwise direction. You step on seven stones in this teaching, within the spirit section of the wheel. Then, as you step from Impeccability to the next stone, you leave the spirit section.

Now you are standing in the south gate. Here you are present in the teachings of the South—in the emotions of your two-legged life. The totem of the South is the coyote. Its element is fire. Its color is green. Its quality is trust and innocence. Its season is summer. Its number is four. Its time is the past. It is a place of dreams and visions and personal feelings. It is the youth of your life, and it is known to be where the plant kingdom is.

Within these teachings of the South, you will be in the presence of your spirit shirt, a coup stick, a vision square, an herb bundle, medicine rocks, a power bundle, a power pouch, a medicine bag, and a dance stick. Within these teachings, you will bring them forth as physical objects. You will be asked to construct these items—things that are given to you to strengthen you in healing your emotions. These are very old teachings, and every teacher has his or her way, just as there are many medicine wheels with many personal teachings.

The Rainbow Medicine Wheel is the personal teaching of myself, Wolf Moondance. I have seen many medicine wheels in my life, and I have heard many teachings and listened to many elders, and I have learned that my vision of the seven stars holds hands with seven points of light that are the lessons within each star. It is within the South that your Clarity must be learned, that you must gain your Poise, attain your Discipline, learn to Account for your actions, know your Fact, make Sense, and be Complete. When this happens you will touch base and stand on the stars of Strength, Success, Vision, Beauty, Healing, Power, and Great.

The vision of the sun, the moon, and the seven stars comes with the offer of sacred teachings that show you a way to listen to your spirit, that show you a way to heal your emotions, that show you a way to respect your physicality and to operate from the fullness of your mind. I open to you the opportunity to find your own vision by listening, by deepening your relationship with the elk, the land turtle, the hawk, the dragonfly, the frog, the owl, and the snake. I offer you now Star Medicine, and hope that it brings a good way to you, that it helps you to walk the good Red Road—the path that is right for you—the right way for you to live, the road of good choices.

Aho.

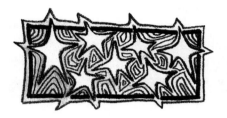

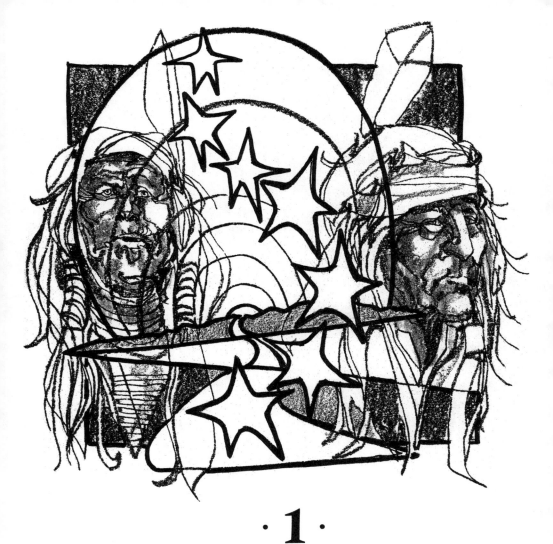

· 1 ·

THE DANCE OF
THE RAINBOW SELF

I breathe in and out, and I relax. I continue breathing deeply, honoring the breath of life that is given to me by Great Spirit. All around me are colors. I see yellows, greens and blues, oranges and reds, purples and burgundies. They are points of light, millions of tiny dots of color. I hear soft singing, the shaking of a rattle, the soft jingling of bells. I hear the big music. It gets larger and larger. I breathe and feel the gentle sway of the soft jingling bells. They are twinkling points of lights. The jingling bells are the songs and the voices of the stars themselves. I smell sweet grass and sage. I smell cedar, a hint of juniper. I smell pine resin and roses. I smell evergreen, the freshness of the forest. I smell the rich dirt of the Earth Mother. As I look out at all the lights, I begin to dance in these colors, and my spirit moves in all directions, in all ways. I feel myself scattering into a million stars. I am all spirit, dancing in whiteness, dancing the rainbow. The colors fill me up—new colors are all around me, shades of purples and turquoises, of teals, corals and salmons, greens and whites, a glistening effervescence. A soft, silvery mist shimmers, moving as smoke. I am that mist. Soft voices sing, "Hao, heyee, heyha." The wind blows the big song through me. The colors swirl, foggy and soft, I am one in spirit with the big music and move to the jingling bells, the clicking rattles, and the soft tap of the drum.

I find myself sitting quietly, leaning against a large rock. I hear thunder rolling across the plains. I feel the intensity of the thunder building in my mind. All around in the prairie grass little flickers of light dart here and there. In front of me seven spirits dance in a circle of color. Moving in pride, they take human form; as two-leggeds they raise their knees high and point their toes. Thunder builds around me. The air is dry and full of ions. I feel the electricity in my hair. I breathe in and out and watch the Dance of the Rainbow Self, the seven spirits prancing around me—in their rich colors—red, orange, yellow, green, blue, purple, and burgundy.

I know them. There is Eagle Woman, one who cries for her heritage, for her knowledge and her existence. And Mouse Hunter, one who seeks fame and to be good enough. There is Tall Woman, the one who has her head in the sky and knows nothing but to keep up with others to hide her own inadequacies. I see Black Horse. I see River Horse. I see Fading Deer and Ghost Sky.

On Mother Earth, where I dwell now as a two-legged, I am a teacher of the Rainbow Dance. I have invited these spirits to walk from their Quest to the thunder of their mind. I have asked them to sit with their emotions and dance the Dance of the Rainbow Self. I have called and they have come. Once again, we open a door. The Medicine Lodge that holds within it the Sacred Circle, the Teaching Lodge, is open. The place where lessons come and medicines are earned. I open up that place for the students—Eagle Woman, Tall Woman, and the others that come—and I see them walking towards the Teaching Lodge, going to the Mystery School, their stories all in place, their emotions thundering and lightning in their minds. The candles are lit in the Sacred Circle—one of each color. I sit in the Teaching

Lodge now, in my mind, listening to their stories. The thunder rolls.

I breathe in and out, and let go. I offer up prayer. I know that Grand-mother, Grandfather, and Great Spirit hear us. "Good evening Grand-mother, Grandfather. Thank you for this opportunity to dance the Rainbow Self. Those who sit here in this Sacred Circle have come to class to listen and to learn. Tell us now, as the soft rain starts to fall, that there is a clearing and a cleansing. Tell us now, Grandmother, Grandfather, your stories of the seven sacred dancers within the Dance of the Rainbow Self. Show us your thoughts that we know as the thunder of our minds, that we call the emotions."

In front of me seven spirits are leaping in the fire of each candle. They are the spirits of the emotions. One dances out. "It is known as Acceptance," Grandmother says.

"There is disgust also," Grandfather says.

There is the emotion of Happy. There is Sad and Anger, and they emerge from the flames. There is Fear and there is Joy. They circle the room and run through the students. The thunder grows and the eagle whistle calls.

A soft green mist surrounds me and I stand in the presence of a pole that is the gateway to the South in the Rainbow Medicine Wheel. I watch the wind blow its flag. When I look around, there is no wheel, just this gateway with the wind blowing the flag, a green cloth. Around the pole are painted seven colors. Around me the green mist spirals, weaves, and turns. First I see only color—bright and clear—swirling, twisting and intertwining—red and green, purple and blue, yellow and orange. They become soft mists, mixing with gold, silver, and white. They are all surrounded by a green tone. They become points of light. And these points become stars. Each one of the stars begins to take the form of an animal. I see the elk, the land turtle, the hawk, then the dragonfly and a frog. There's an owl and a snake. I see a hummingbird, an otter. There is a butterfly, a slug, a weasel, a whale, and a shark. As the colors become stars, the stars become the animal world—the crawlies, the four-legged, the winged-ones. The animals speak and they become words, Great Spirit's words. I hear Strength and Success, Vision and Beauty, Healing and Power, and Great. There is Clarity and Poise, Discipline, Account, Fact, Sense, and Complete. The words become stars again, and colors, but I can see animal faces within it all. The fourteen words, the fourteen stars, the fourteen animals, and the crawlies and winged ones. They are intermixed, in a soft green mist.

I feel myself become one with all of it. Before me I see a small campfire and sitting there is an old, old, old woman. I see the fire reflecting in her face. She is part wolf. Ah, I know this old woman. I hurry toward her. It is

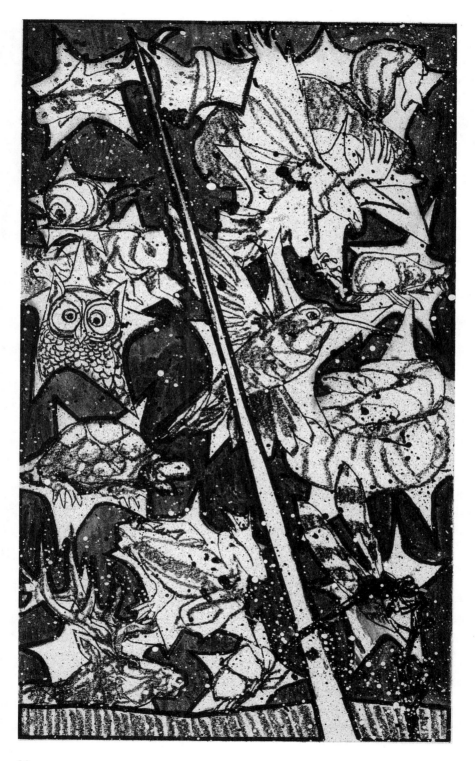

Grandmother Wolf! She's a friendly family member.

"Grandmother, let me tell you what I've seen!"

She looks at me and she says, "Beware. Be careful. There is trickery. Be careful—in the thunder and lightning there is rage and hate. Don't you understand, dear?"

I watch her poke the fire. She takes out a little rattle and starts shaking it. Then she gets up and dances around the fire. "Be careful. There is danger. Don't you understand?"

I see the worried look in her face. "It's hard. It's hard for me to understand, Grandmother. You know so much more than I do."

"No, I don't know any more than you. You need to be quiet and listen. You need to understand that the emotions are much more powerful than the body. That they have the ability to speak through the mind. They have a way of ruling your life. Be careful, Granddaughter." She stokes up the fire and the little tiny sparks flicker in the air. They spin around and I see colors in each one of the sparks.

"Grandmother, all I can see are the sparks, and when I see the sparks, I see the same thing I've been seeing. I see these colors and I see these fourteen spirits. They speak to me of medicines—they say they're medicines—seven of them, and they say they're lessons, seven of them."

"It is your vision, Granddaughter." She puts another log on the fire and sits on the old stump. She looks at me with a softness in her yellow eyes, and she says, "It is the ancient wisdom that we have here within us that allows us to remember our spirit. We must remember to be in balance, Granddaughter.

"These students you have, they are following the path. They are walking, and every day that they walk, there is a hardness to life. There are many obstacles, sadness, and disgust. There are big obstacles these people face—big fears. They fear starving to death. They fear the pain of dying. They become angry and live in discord."

"Grandmother, I've become quite comfortable walking the path, carrying the vision with me."

"Oh, don't become complacent," she says. "Look at the earth and it will tell you the story of sadness. You'll see the beauty of green everywhere. Let me share with you something, now. Let me prepare you, Granddaughter. Red is Acceptance. Acceptance is red. Orange is Disgust. Disgust is orange. Yellow is Happy. Happy is yellow. Green is sad. Sad is green. Blue is Anger. Anger is blue. Fear is purple. Purple is fear. Joy is burgundy and burgundy Joy. Before they were words they were colors.

"Long ago, in the beginning, before the two-legged, there was only the thought of Great Spirit. Grandmother, Grandfather, Great Spirit. When I was just a pup I remember. I remember quietly listening to Great Spirit, Grandmother, Grandfather talk, talking of the feelings, great armies of emotions—great gatherings of feelings. I would look at what Grandfather and Grandmother pointed at and I would see a swirling mass of color. I would know it to be feelings. There they were, each one of them. A red one, a green one, a blue one. Everything is color.

"I tell you, the seven primary emotions are what I speak of. And I tell you their colors. Many lies are told—that Anger is red, for example."

"I can see that, Grandmother. I can see how red would be Anger. I can see it. Full of fire, burning deep inside of you, Grandmother."

"No, people say that Anger is red because they judge it by how it feels. Anger burns and destroys so often that it is lied about. They say that the color of Anger is red because it is like fire. Isn't that funny? Because fire isn't red," Grandmother says.

"Well, I guess fire looks red and it burns, so Anger would be like fire and be red," I say.

"But, Granddaughter, fire is yellow and orange, white and blue. Anger is blue—it is so hot it is cold—and as blue is cold, so is Anger."

"But anger is red—and that is hot," I say.

"No, Granddaughter, Acceptance is red. Being strong enough, having your Strength, is Acceptance. The two-legged don't remember clearly. They forget their Clarity and lose their Acceptance. And they stand there, naked, in Disgust. You know, here on the Earth Mother we are the children."

She stokes the fire and the flame belches higher. It lights up the sky with a golden orange tone. We're sitting on top of a mesa, in the middle of openness. One shake at a time she rattles a deer bone hollowed out and filled with stones. "Crystals, to be exact," she says. They click and rattle against the dry bone. "Granddaughter, be careful! These seven spirits, they are the primary emotions and all two-leggeds have them. It is from the South that our emotions are known. You must remember the coyote. You must study carefully the ways of the coyote."

"Well, Grandmother, many say that the coyote is playful, and youthful."

"Oh, yes, Granddaughter. It is. In the South is the summertime, a time of youth. You know, they say 'to make hay . . .' But there are many, many feelings and many, many emotions. That's why you see so many points of light, Granddaughter. They are your primary lights, the ones that you see the strongest. These are known as the bold colors. Then there are the secondary colors, the ones you don't pay much attention to. They're feelings that are just there—that you don't do much about.

"Then there are your tri-levels. Those are the feelings that you can't get to go away. Those are the ones that persist, move on, and charge ahead—they're more complicated—not simple words. Then there are your faceted ones, the fourth level, the totality of the mind. Emotions at their deepest level, like rage and hate, love and jealousy, insanity . . . sanity."

She puts her head back and softly laughs. "Ha, ha, ha, ha. You see, the two-leggeds never quite get it all figured out. They forget this formula, that first comes color, then the misty movement swirling about becomes a star as matter collects into its form. Its first form was that of the animal in us all, our primal, our cellular memory that brings forth our humanness, which is simply an illusion of death. It is the last phase of the mammal, the animal—it is the last phase of the warm-blooded and the cold-blooded, before we all become just a word. Great Spirit's words, all of them. Evil and good." The fire belches and the sparks fly high in the sky. She pulls back from the fire and looks at me. "You're fading, Granddaughter. Be careful, your thoughts are weak. I warned you of your emotions."

Then in a flash of lightning she is gone, and I'm sitting and looking at the seven colors in human reality, flickering in the night lodge, the Teaching Lodge, where Tall Woman, Mouse Hunter, River Horse, and others have gathered to hear the lessons of *why*, to find out the secrets, to understand their childhood, to understand today and tomorrow. To grasp the great secrets of life.

"Remember, Granddaughter, it's dangerous here within the emotions. The beauty is within the dance itself. Before you lie seven doorways, seven stars of medicine that treat the seven lessons. Each student here and those who lie beyond want to know why they do what they do, why did they do what they did, why they will do what they will do. Be careful, Granddaughter! Be careful, Granddaughter!"

I hear the soft sounds of the stars calling me back.

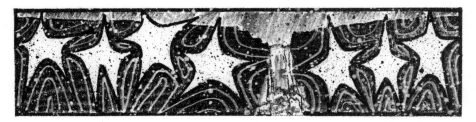

The words that you read here are real. Strength lives as a medicine in this section of the medicine wheel known as Rainbow Medicine. It is an application of Fact, Complete, dance and emotion. Within Star Medicine you are opening yourself up to the companionship, the accountability, the dedication, the responsibility, and the sincerity of the southern section of the wheel. You are stepping into the South. Maybe it's your first time working with the medicine wheel. Maybe it's your first time walking with the teachings of shamanism. There are ways to do things that are known to be sacred. Any time that you work with ceremonial tools such as herbs, they are medicines. When you work with prayer, it is a medicine. When you work with lessons, they are a medicine. You may need to use candles, prayers, prayer ties, prayer beads, prayer lines, rocks, skins, cloth, which are known as sacred tools. All those things lie ahead of you. They are there to assist you. They are there to help you translate and understand the words of Great Spirit.

I will offer you many important messages in these pages. The first is "Set your home in a sacred way." That means to clean out all the bad. Remove the bad memories; remove the bad people; remove the bad situations. Understand that working with the emotions is very powerful, and there are going to be a lot of feelings. I recommend that your home be a place of safety. If it's not, then bring it forth. Don't let your life be taken away from you by someone else's angers or someone else's fears. Open up your place, bring forth your home. Get your ceremonial tools, have your herbs and your scents; have your smells, your places, and let your objects be yours. Don't allow anything or anyone to take away your sacredness, for within your emotions is your knowing. Understand that your sacred tools and your sacred place, your spirit journal, and the ceremonies you learn in this book are a gift now, in this time. I have learned these ways through many years in shamanism, working with nature and what is natural, with humans and spirits, that you may relate to Great Spirit, Creator, God, and have a rich, full, human spiritual experience.

Ceremony of Smudging

Smudging is a ceremony that cleans and balances. You do it with burning herbs that bring forth smoke. Smoke is a communication with Great Spirit. The herb sage represents your prayers. You can also use tobacco to smudge, or sweet grass, or other healing herbs, such as osha root or bitter root, but what is usually used is sweet grass or sage.

Place your prayer in the herb by thinking very carefully and communicating clear thoughts of balance. "Balance" means being refreshed—the old has been understood, and now is now, a new day is a new way. Balance means honoring—taking time to see things the way they are, not the way you want or need them to be, but the way they are, honored by your understanding and going on with a good and solid feeling. Balance means respecting—knowing that all of life is Great Spirit, and that each time we respect we are in balance. Respect is applying the knowing that we have a choice in what we see. When we respect, we choose to see anything and all things as good and light, knowing the bad is our other choice. To bring good to all things in life is sometimes hard, but we give respect when we do it. Then the boundary of good is set as our point and our point is Great Spirit, and all our actions will be built up of positive energy. The smudging ceremony then cleans and balances our energy, making us ready for any ceremonial work we are going to do.

You will need a bowl. I recommend an abalone shell—you can often find one at a rock shop or health food store if not at the beach—for it is the right size to hold the herbs, but you can use anything that is not going to catch on fire, such as clay, marble, or alabaster. The bowl represents the earth and the fire that lights the herbs represents the cleansing. The smoke represents the carrying of the prayers. Your prayers are transformed into smoke and are carried to Great Spirit.

In this process, you light the sage or whatever herb you are using. As it starts to smoke, start at the bottom of your body, around your feet, and using your hand or a feather, fan in a clockwise motion, working upwards and around you. Work behind you by placing the bowl behind your body, using your other hand to move the smoke up and around your body. Lift it up over your head, and all over the outer portions of your body to cleanse your aura. Your outer energy fields are here, and they must be kept balanced at all times. When the outer energy field is cleansed and balanced, this helps the alignment of the inner energy fields that are your center, keeping you in balance. Think of your body as made of feathers or fur. As you cleanse yourself see the smoke stroking you and removing anything that might be catching in your hair, on your fur, feathers, or skin. You are actually removing negative ions and replacing them with positive ions, which are balancing the forces of energy around your body. It is important for your ions to be positive and high, to keep your body in a healthy and good way.

Smudging is also done to cleanse your tools. You need to smudge all things before using them, before taking them into a ceremony or before giving them to anyone. Again, light a bowl full of herbs. Run the object through the smoke four times. Then turn it over and run it through four more times, making sure that you have made four complete circles twice, for a total of eight times. This honors the entire wheel of seven medicines and the center, which is Creator.

Smudging is a ceremony of balance, respect, rejuvenation, and refreshment. It is meant to bring things into balance—"things" being not only objects but also the energy around you. And remember that herbs are the oldest medicines in physical form.

Aho.

Spirit Journal

I recommend journaling because it is a personal expression in physical form. I recommend it because it can open doors for you. Your journal is a place where you put your private thoughts, a place where there are no rules and no expectations. It is a safety zone where you can express your feelings.

Sometimes you may be afraid to put your feelings on paper because other people will intrude on your space. It is very wrong for anyone to read another person's spirit journal without its owner's permission. When people's curiosity crosses over the line and takes them into the private space of the spirit journal, it can be grounds for termination of the connection, be it blood kin, good friend, or otherwise. The Native way is to give your word. When men, women, or children give their word, that is all that is necessary. It is important to have your privacy, a place where you can write down your feelings of Anger, Joy, Fear, Acceptance—all the emotions—without being afraid that someone is going to hold them against you or use them against you. If this is the case, your spirit journal will allow you to end that relationship. It is important to terminate relationships when your trust has been violated.

So my Wolf advice—"Wolf" meaning guardian, parent, or teacher—is that each of us must respect each other's space, and a spirit journal is a good place to start. It is also a give-away, a gift, something that stays behind long after you have died. It is an object you leave for your friends, your children, your loved ones, so that they can look back and see how you struggled or stood solid, how you thought things through, how you really did care—or you didn't care. I recommend a spirit/personal journal in all of my writings, in all levels of the medicine wheel—so that you can keep up with things, so that you can record your venturing forth in your own quest. If you have a teacher, it is a good place to put your assignments, like the ceremonies and the processes that I have placed in these books. I am your personal teacher in this book. When you do my exercises or follow my requests, then you are following my guidance and your spirit journal will hold the things you need to remember. Sometimes you get lost in the rush of your daily life and forget what your objective or your intention is. Then your journal is there to guide you back to the right path. It is a good place to write down your intentions and your objectives and bring forth your path for yourself.

To prepare a journal, you need a notebook of a color that represents your emotions, which would be green. You can color it, you can glue things on it, you can bead it, cover it with leather or glitter, put pictures on it—you can do just about anything you want to, to bring it forth as a personal journal. It is a good idea to keep a rainbow on the front so that you know that you are walking with all seven medicines. When you personalize the outside of your journal, you make it yours—the home of your sacred writings, where you examine your emotions, your memories, your dreams, your visions, your conversations with the spirit world, your animal guides, and everything that is true for you in the south part of the medicine wheel.

Your journal will keep everything in it about Star Medicine, which *is* your emotions. The stars speak to you in your journal. You can record things in it that help keep your thoughts clear and in order.

You can write in your journal what we call a 1-25. A 1-25 is a list of things that you are going to do on the next day. The night before, you make a list in your journal of everything that you want to do. You then bring this list out and follow it the next day.

When you are not using your spirit journal, keep it in a sacred traveling case, or wrap it in red cotton cloth, and place it inside another object, such as a medicine bag, purse, or briefcase that you carry with you. Your respect for your spirit journal is very important, for it teaches you to respect yourself.

A lot of people want to do the exercises in this book, but find it hard. Adding the exercises and journaling to your 1-25 list will help get these things done. You could put all these exercises in your book.

Example: I will sit for 15 minutes and do the exercise on journaling. I will simply take out my journal, open it, date it, and write down my feelings today. I will try to express myself on 1) Acceptance, how I feel about Acceptance; 2) how I feel about Disgust: something that disgusted me today; 3) how I feel about Happiness: something that made me happy today; 4) what made me Sad; 5) what made me angry: how did I get

Angry today—what brought it about? 6) what was my Fear: what did I fear today? Here I list all my fears for the day; and 7) what brought me Joy?

Another interesting exercise or conversation for your journal is to explore the depth of Joy, write the definitions, what other people have told you it is, and what you know it to be, and expand on it that way.

Your journal will be a rewarding experience. You will reach a point where your Fears are understood; your Angers are understood; your Sadness is understood; your Happiness is expanded upon, and the things that Disgust you are dealt with. You will find it a process from which you will gather great rewards in the days to come.

Ceremony of Prayer Ties

Tools: *Cloth or soft, colored paper (like napkins); tobacco; red yarn; a blanket; sage and sweet grass for smudging; smudge bowl, matches; plus extra sage and sweet grass, and cornmeal.*

Making a prayer tie is actually making a prayer. The first thing you do is lay out a blanket on which to sit to do your work. If you choose, this can become your medicine blanket, which contains the energies of all your work. This can be a place where you sit with your prayers, or it can be where you place your prayers.

You will then want to cut the cloth or colored paper. You can use whatever color you wish to use, but I recommend 100% red cotton cloth or blue cotton cloth, if you choose to do your prayer ties in cloth. You cut the cloth into one-inch (2.5 cm) squares. Prepare the square piece of cloth or paper by laying it flat. Then take a pinch of tobacco, sweet grass, sage, and cornmeal—or simple tobacco, or simply sweet grass and sage—if you choose not to work with tobacco, and place it in the center of the square. Then pull the corners up, gather them, and tie them with red yarn around the top, making a pinch bundle. There is no required number of prayers other than to make one prayer a day, but I usually ask that my students make prayers in fours or sevens to represent the four directions or the seven sacred teachings. You can also do discipline prayer numbers by setting a number of prayers each day that you wish to make.

Once your prayer ties are done, tie them together on a string or yarn, making a line. Wrap the line on a stick and place the stick in a fire that you have built outside and let the smoke carry the prayers to the Great Spirit. Or you can hang the line in a tree by draping it along the branches and letting the deer come and nourish themselves on the prayers, carrying the prayers to Great Spirit. The deer is a carrier of prayer, as are the rain and the sunshine.

You may also choose to place the prayer ties on a prayer line around your medicine wheel. Simply place a stick in the ground every so often around the wheel and tie the line from stick to stick until you have made a total circle. Then drape the prayers on the lines around the wheel.

Working with your prayers gives you a feeling of accomplishment. You realize that your prayer is not an unheard or unfelt commodity. When you work with prayer ties, it gives you a chance to connect your prayers to the colors. If, for example, you are tying prayers for Strength, you would tie red prayer ties. If you are tying prayers for the Spirit, you would tie red prayer ties. If you are tying prayers for Success, you would tie them in orange. It's okay to think of a topic and make your own choice of color, for within Rainbow Medicine there is no wrong. You can create prayer ties for many things, and the best way to understand how to use Rainbow Medicine is to pray about it and think about where the subject would be in the medicine wheel.

If you wanted to make prayer ties about sexual things, for example, sexual would be physical—a physical act; therefore, you would go to the physical part of the wheel which is blue, which is in the West, and you would tie blue prayer ties. This would also bring about the truth, for blue is about truth.

If you were going to make prayer ties about love, love being an emotional and mental thing, you would make them in green and white. They would be in the emotional section *and* in the physical section. Or, you could look at the word *love* and see it as power, and make purple prayer ties. It's important that you connect your own personal words to the colors and make your prayers in that way. If you are using white, you are always praying for something spiritual, tying prayers from the mind, from the soul, from the North, from the spirit. If you are using black, then you are praying for wholeness and totality, making prayers ties to give yourself a place to stand in your completeness. It would be your totality or your wholeness that you'd be praying about—these are the only words that I use black for. No negative prayer ties can be made in this program. Your prayer ties cannot be used for selfish purposes or in hate.

When you have finished your prayer ties, it is important to let go of the thoughts you have placed inside them. You were thinking clearly when you made the prayer tie, but for prayer to be honest, you need to let go and release the idea, knowing it is energy of Great Spirit now.

Place your prayer ties on the prayer lines at your medicine wheel or on the ground around the outside of the medicine wheel, or tie them in a tree to release them and let them go to Great Spirit.

On the solstices it is very important that you remove all prayer ties from trees or prayer lines and put them in a fire, releasing the prayers and allowing them to be carried to Grandfather, Grandmother, Great Spirit. You could also do this on the full moon of each month. Or you can burn them only on the night of the solstices. Burning your prayers is a release of the physical form of the prayer and is a Discipline.

If you live in a place where you have no trees to hang your prayer ties on, you need to find someone who will give you permission to hang the prayer lines in their trees. If you cannot find a place where you can build a fire, I suggest burying the prayer ties in order to release them. You could also mail them to someone who can hang them, burn them, or bury them.

Building a Rainbow Medicine Wheel and Using the Green Section

These are instructions for building an outside wheel that is large enough for you to move around in. If you don't have enough space to build a wheel this big, you can build a smaller indoor or outdoor wheel in the same way—just decrease the size of the rocks and the poles. When you use a small wheel, you perform the ceremony sitting outside the wheel, looking into it. When you use a large wheel, you actually go inside the gates and move around inside the wheel. You can sit on one of the rocks, one that represents what you wish to study.

Tools: *Rocks, poles, flags, white votive candles, clay or shell candle holders; red yarn or cords, smudging tools. All these tools are described in detail here.*

1. Gather the rocks and cleanse them (page 32).
   a) Find a center point for your wheel. It can be a buffalo skull or a large crystal, a blue-painted rock, or a blue rock, but it must be large—

bigger than a human head. The center represents Great Spirit, Creator, God. It can also be a small fire pit, about 8 to 10 inches (20 to 25 cm) across. The fire will represent Great Spirit.

b) **Song Rocks.** You'll need seven rocks that are a little smaller, about half the size of the Creator stone. Each one of these rocks is a different color—red, orange, yellow, green, blue, purple, and burgundy. They can be painted. They represent the Song and the seven stars. They make up the first circle around the Creator stone.

c) **Direction Rocks.** You'll need four rocks that are smaller than the Creator rock, but larger than the Song Rocks. Each one needs to be one of the following colors—red, green, blue, and white. The red rock represents spirit in the East, the green represents emotions in the South, the blue represents the body in the West, and the white represents the mind in the North.

   The rocks can be those colors naturally, or you can paint them. If you like, you can paint them with symbols that you have chosen to represent the four directions in those four colors.

d) **Star Rocks—Medicine Rocks.** You'll need seven medicine rocks for each direction—that's four sets of seven stones. Each set of seven stones is a full rainbow. On each is painted one of the seven colors to represent its special medicine. For example, in the red group (the East) you would have a red rock, or a rock with a red star or a red symbol painted on it. You would also have an orange rock in the red series, and a yellow, a green, a blue, a purple, and a burgundy rock. In the green (the South), you would do it the same way. In the blue (the West), the same, and in the white (the North), also—28 stones altogether. These are your Medicine Rocks for the four directions.

   Each medicine has its own symbol, but in the medicine wheel I use the symbol of the star to represent this group. Place these rocks starting in the East and moving clockwise around the circle. The seven rocks in the red series go from the east stone to the south stone; the seven rocks in the green series go from the south to the west stone; the seven rocks in the blue series go from the west to the north stone, and the seven rocks in the white series go from the North to the East, completing the circle.

e) **Lesson Rocks.** You'll need seven lesson rocks for each of the four directions—28 rocks in all. Start with a plain rock. The spirit section gets a red circle painted on each rock. Then paint a solid dot of color inside each circle. This dot should be in the lesson color—red, orange, yellow, green, blue, purple, and burgundy.

Example: red (or color of direction)
            solid-colored dot in color of lesson

Each section works the same way. The outer circle is the color of the direction: Red is the East, the section of the spirit. Green is the South, the section of the emotions. Blue is the West, the section of the body; and white is the North, the section of the mind.

All the lesson dots are the seven colors—red, orange, yellow, green, blue, purple, burgundy. You can personalize each stone with your own symbol instead of a dot, if you want. Keep your symbols simple and basic, using color and light and good concepts, such as animals, plants, minerals, and elements.

Make sure the paint you use is waterproof and won't wash off.

When you place the Lesson Stones, lay them from the gate stone to the center stone.

Example: The Direction Rocks are on the right, left, top, and bottom of the wheel, and the center is the Creator stone. The seven Lesson Stones are placed in a straight line from the gate stone to the center—right to left, left to right, top to center, bottom to center, so that they form a cross with the Creator stone in the middle.

It's a good idea to wash the rocks before you prepare to paint them. Do that with fresh water from a garden hose, or place them in the ocean, a lake or creek or in any running water. After you wash the rocks, allow them to sun dry. Let this take place over one full day. When the rocks have dried, they will be cleansed of any activities that have gone on before. Move the rocks through the smudge smoke four times each. It is now time to paint them, put symbols on them, or get them ready to be identified with the direction.

2. **Preparing the gates.**
   a) **Poles.** You'll need 12 poles. Eight of them should be five to seven feet (1.5–2m) tall. Four of them should be three to five feet (1–1.5m) tall. They can be of any type of wood, preferably limbs that have fallen from trees naturally. Driftwood would be good. Or you can use wooden poles that you buy at the lumberyard. These poles become your gates. You have one at the East, made with two of the tall poles; a gateway to the South, made with two of the tall poles; and the same with the West and the North. Then you place the four shorter center poles in the southeast, the southwest, the northwest, and the northeast.

b) **Flags, candles, and yarn.** You'll need four colored flags, red for the East, green for the South, blue for the West and white for the North, plus four candles in the same colors, and red yarn for the prayer lines.

3. Start the ceremony of building the wheel. First select the ground on which you want your medicine wheel to be built. This should be a private spot where you won't be intruded upon by people, distracting or excessive noise, animals or children running and playing. Or you can choose to build it indoors in a very quiet, undisturbed place inside your apartment or home. It is not necessary to build a medicine wheel outdoors, but it is much more effective in natural surrounding.

One of the best locations is beside water—near a pond, a lake, or an ocean. Choose an area that is open to the sky, where the energy can move down from the sky to the ground. The place where you build your medicine wheel is up to you. It will become a sacred space, a sacred circle, a place for you to go for the spiral of energy that will strengthen your spirit.

The spot you choose should be clean and raked, washed or swept. It can be plain dirt, but the dirt should be healthy. It can be grassy. It can be sand. Or it can have carpet or be hardwood, if it is indoors. A family wheel is eight feet (2.5m) in diameter. A community wheel is sixteen feet (5m) in diameter. A personal wheel is four feet or two feet (1.2–.6m) in diameter. It is important, if you are building a wheel inside a tepee, that you have the top open, so smoke can go out through the top, and so that the center is open to the sky. If you are building the wheel in a room, be sure you have it where there is a cross direction of two windows, so that air can move through the room from one side to the other, and come and go, and where light can be present.

4. Start the Ceremony. First, honor the ground by giving prayer and a give-away of sage, cornmeal, tobacco, sweet grass. Do this by pinching and breaking off the sage and sweet grass, taking a pinch of tobacco and cornmeal, and holding it up towards the sky, honoring Great Spirit for allowing you to do this ceremony. Then hold the herbs down towards the earth, to honor Mother Earth, that she is there for you to have the ceremony upon. Honor the four directions by holding the herbs out to the spirit in the East and thanking the spirit for coming. Honor the South, the emotions, for being there and letting you feel. Hold the herbs towards the West and honor the West for allowing you to have the body to do this ceremony with. Hold them to the North and honor the North for giving you the mind for doing this ceremony.

Then hold the herbs towards your left shoulder and drop them onto the ground, offering prayers for the spirits—all the spirits that will come to your wheel, all the subjects, the guardians, and present forms of spirit. Only ask for what you want to have come, and for knowledge from the medicines and lessons. Smudge the area by fanning the smoke with your hand in an upright motion. This begins the ceremony of the medicine wheel.

5. Place the stones. When you have placed your honoring and your respect ceremony of tobacco, cornmeal, sweet grass, and sage on the ground, find the center of your wheel, a place where you know your wheel begins. This will be a very powerful spot. In it you will face the East, and honor it. Face the South, and honor it. Face the West, and honor it. Face the North, and honor it. While you do this, hold in your hands the stone that will be the center, the buffalo skull, or the objects to build a fire pit. Then place the center.

Gather seven Song Rocks to make the circle around the center. Holding them one at a time, step to the center and turn to face the East and place the red stone. Then move a little clockwise towards the South, and place the orange. Move a little bit more and place the yellow. Facing due South you will place the green stone. Moving a little bit, place the blue stone. Move a little more and place the purple stone and a little bit more, and place the burgundy stone. Then look at the circle around the center and space out the stones evenly so that they are placed all the way around. You have now brought forth the center, the representation of Great Spirit, and the singing—the song of life.

As you place your rocks, never turn around—always move forward. When you turn around, you break the energy. Move clockwise as you place the rocks. Never pick one up and move it with your hand once you have set it in its position, as this would show that you feel inadequate about yourself, that you feel you have done something wrong. There is no wrong in the medicine wheel. Keep going clockwise, moving the rocks with your foot until you get them right where you want them.

Now for the larger stones that you have selected for the four directions. Start in the East and place the large red stone. This rock represents the spirit. Step seven feet (2m) out from the balance point between the yellow and the green Song Rocks in the center, and place the green rock. This is the south gate. Stepping off just a little from the green Song Rock, pace out seven feet and set the blue stone; this is the west gate. Walking on around and facing the south rock, looking straight across at the green rock, you then set down the north stone, a white rock.

RAINBOW MEDICINE WHEEL

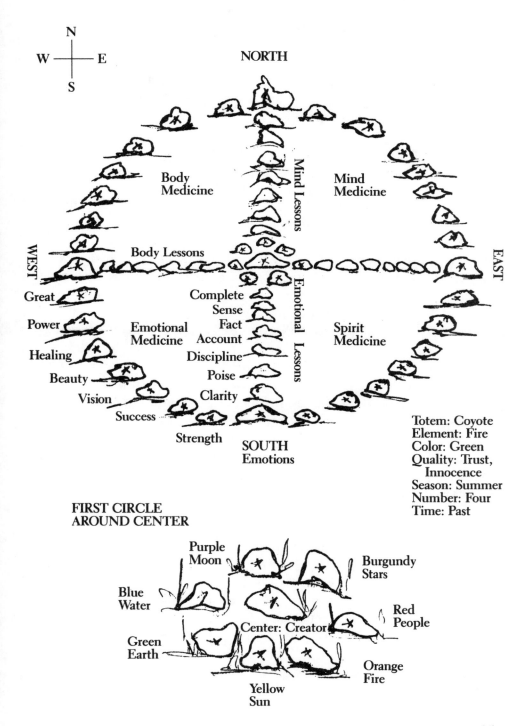

N
W — E
S

NORTH

Body Medicine

Mind Lessons

Mind Medicine

WEST

Body Lessons

EAST

Great
Power
Healing
Beauty
Vision
Success
Strength

Emotional Medicine

Complete
Sense
Fact
Account
Discipline
Poise
Clarity

Emotional Lessons

Spirit Medicine

SOUTH
Emotions

Totem: Coyote
Element: Fire
Color: Green
Quality: Trust,
    Innocence
Season: Summer
Number: Four
Time: Past

FIRST CIRCLE
AROUND CENTER

Purple
Moon
Blue
Water
Green
Earth
Yellow
Sun

Center: Creator

Burgundy
Stars
Red
People
Orange
Fire

35

When you have placed the four directions, it is time to set down your medicine stones. These are your Star Rocks. Starting at the East and working clockwise towards the South, place the stones to form an arc in that section. You will then honor the South by stepping over the south stone and placing an arc of seven medicine stones in the next section. You will then step over the west stone, honoring the West, and place the arc representing the body, the West. Then, stepping over the north stone, the white one, you will place an arc of seven stones representing the North, the mind. When you have placed these 28 stones, you will have all four directions of medicines, and you will return to the east stone.

Remember never to turn around and move counterclockwise, which would create negative energy. Always move clockwise.

You will be looking towards the center. Stepping off towards the center, you will place red, orange, yellow, green, blue, purple, and burgundy stones, representing the lessons. The burgundy stone will be right outside the center, close to the red stone of the Song. Then move down, honor the south stone and the south gate, turn and face the center. Place the next seven Lesson Stones, from the outside in towards the center, red through burgundy. When you have placed the burgundy stone, honor the center and move to the West. Standing with your heels at the blue stone, face the center and lay down the Lesson Stones for the West: red, orange, yellow, green, blue, purple, burgundy. Then, honoring the center, turn and move to the North. Honor the North, turn and place your heels against the north stone. Lay down the last seven Lesson Stones, red through burgundy. You have now placed your Lesson Stones. Give thanks for the lessons that will come. Now walk to the east gate and exit the wheel.

When you look back you will see the center rock with seven Song Rocks around it, four large direction stones, a medicine circle of four sets of seven, and a cross in the center that forms four sets of seven. Your medicine stones are now in place.

Remember, when moving in the wheel and placing stones, always to move clockwise, the direction of positive energy.

6. **Place the poles.** Stand in the East, behind the east stone, and face the outside of the wheel. Take two large steps and dig a hole in the ground on each side of you. Place one of the tall poles in each hole, burying the ends deep in the ground so that the poles are solid. They will form a gate large enough for you to walk through. Then move to the South and do the same thing. Repeat these movements, stepping back two feet (.6m), digging holes and placing the gates, until you have two tall poles in the East, two in the

South, two in the West and two in the North. Move on clockwise to the East. Staying outside the circle, step to the center space between the east and the south rocks. There you need to dig a hole and place the shorter southeast pole. Move to the South and in the center space between the south and the west rocks, dig a hole and place the pole. Move to the West and in the center between the west and the north rocks, dig a hole and place a pole. Move to the North and, between the north and the east rocks, dig a hole and place the northeast pole. Now you have formed a circle of poles around the medicine wheel, on the outside of the rocks.

7. **Tie the cords.** Return to the gateway of the East. Standing in the East, face the center and tie the red yarn or cord to the left pole of the east gate. Moving clockwise, wrap the cord around the center (the shorter) pole and then move on to the right-hand pole of the south gate, facing the center. Tie it off and cut it, so that you leave the gate open. Now tie a string to the left-hand-side pole of the south gate; walk on clockwise and wrap it around the center (shorter) pole; and then move to the right-hand side of the west pole, and tie it off. Leaving the gateway open, tie the cord to the left-hand pole and move on clockwise, wrapping it around the center pole, and tying it to the right-hand pole of the north gate. Cut the cord, and leaving the north gate open, tie the cord to the left-hand side of the north gate. Walk on clockwise and wrap the cord around the center pole and tie it to the right-hand-side pole of the east gate. You will now be standing on the outside of the wheel, looking through the gateway to the center of the wheel.

Looking at the wheel now, you'll see that you have tied lines that form a complete circle, but have left all four gates open. You can attach your prayer ties to these lines.

Always enter and leave the medicine wheel through the east gate, moving clockwise around the wheel. Only spirits use the other gates—not two-leggeds. As you enter, it is important to face the West and to allow the chief spirit of the medicine wheel, the Bear, to move through the medicine wheel. When you leave the east, south, west, and north gates open, you are asking ancestor spirits to enter. Your spirit, along with the spirits of the East, enter through the East and carry your body inside the medicine wheel.

The medicine wheel is a very sacred place. Do not do anything inside your medicine wheel that would bring offense to Great Spirit. There should be no anger or disturbance, and no liquor or drugs used inside a medicine wheel.

8. **Place the candles.** When you have the Rainbow Medicine Wheel

built, stand at the east gate. Have four votive candles in glass votive-type candle holders, and wooden matches. Kneel at the east gate and place a red candle on top of or beside the east rock. Then enter into the medicine wheel, raise your hands to the sky, and shake them gently to honor Grandmother, Grandfather spirits. Turn to the East and light the candle. Move to the South and place a green candle on the ground or on the south rock. Light it, rise, and honor the South. Move to the West and place a blue candle on the ground or on the west rock, light it, rise, and honor the West. Move to the North and place a white candle on the ground, or on the rock. Light it, rise, and honor the North.

Honoring—unless I have specified another way to go about it—usually means to raise your hands and shake them gently. This acknowledges the spirit. You may also spin around in a complete circle, signifying that your whole body has acknowledged the spirit of each direction.

If you are setting the candle on the ground, only place it on dirt. Do not put it where anything can catch fire. Be responsible within your wheel. Its power is very strong and it teaches many lessons.

Move to the East, for now you will walk into the wheel to the center. Light a white candle in honor of Great Spirit, Grandfather, Grandmother, giving prayers of thanks for bringing forth the vision of the sun, the moon, and the seven stars. Place it in the center as you give thanks to the Mother Wheel, the Rainbow Medicine Wheel, where you will have the song of Great Spirit, Grandmother, Grandfather. Then place a candle beside each one of the Song Rocks—the red, orange, yellow, green, blue, purple, and burgundy—to honor your song. Place them in the center inside the Song Rocks. The candles must match the colors of the stones. When you place the red candle, it is in honor of the people. When you place the orange candle, it is in honor of fire. When you place the yellow candle, it is in honor of the sun. When you place the green candle, it is in honor of the earth. When you place the blue candle, it is in honor of the water. When you place the purple candle, it is in honor of the moon. And when you place the burgundy candle, it is in honor of the stars. Light your candles, moving clockwise, and return to the East.

9. **Place the flags.** To finish your medicine wheel, place a red flag on the left pole of the east gate. When you tie this flag around the pole, the gate is open for the wind spirits to come and go. Place a green flag on the left pole of the south gate, a blue flag on the left pole of the west gate, and a white flag on the left pole of the north gate. These flags proclaim that the gates are open, that the lessons, the medicines, and the teachings of the spirits are

brought forth, and that the medicine of each direction may come and go. Your wheel is now open to enjoy and to bring forth a memory that we are always a part of the Rainbow Medicine Wheel. All people are welcome in this wheel—all races, all religions, all creeds, for we are all one within the Rainbow Medicine Wheel.

Remember, the medicine wheel is a symbol of totality. You never step out of a medicine wheel; you only step out of a symbol.

Using the Medicine Wheel

You can use the wheel at any time of the day or the year. East corresponds to the springtime; South to the summer; West to the fall; North to the winter. You can sit in the appropriate section of those times of year.

As for time of day, East is the morning; South is the afternoon; West is the evening, and North is night. You can move around your wheel according to the time of day.

Remember when you are in the wheel that you will hear and see and feel everything that is necessary. You never need to feel pushed or that you are missing something. If you let your thoughts go, then you will know. The voice and teachings of spirit will come through your mind.

It is important that you journal what you hear. Anything.

Example: *You are sitting in the south part of the wheel to study your emotions. It is noontime of a summer day. You are listening, and you hear a simple sentence: "You can do it." After that you see a flag waving in the breeze with a dragonfly over it. It is important that you write all this down in your journal, for you have received the message that all things are possible at noontime, in the summer, for you. You can fulfill your dream, for a dragonfly signified a dream. Write down the color of the flag. Let's say it was blue. You would turn to the lesson words and the medicine words in the back of the book, and you would know that you are going to receive a healing, for the blue word is "healing" in the medicine section. Then you would look at the lesson words, and you'd know that the lesson you are learning would be Fact, so you'd know that this is a fact.*

All you need to do is sit and listen to what is said to you. Do not try to force things. Do not make believe that something is happening when it isn't—*it will happen.* While you never need to force it, never say to yourself, "Oh, well, it's just my imagination." Your imagination is your gateway to the spirit and the voice of your spirit comes through your imagination, allowing you to find your answers.

Everything in your life of emotions is based on spirit, and your physical body is based on emotions. Looking at the medicine wheel as a physical location, it is a place to feel, see, learn, and converse with yourself and others in a good way. You yourself are a sacred wheel, and all of your life is the medicine wheel. As you study the Rainbow Medicine Wheel, you can simplify your life to the 28 medicines and 28 lessons. As you practice and study the words, you will expand to a deeper level of life. The medicine wheel is a place where you can share feeling and listen to what you hear in your mind, communicating with the spirits within the wheel. That is the whole purpose of building a medicine wheel. It is very sacred.

It's a good idea to bring bird feed to the medicine wheel and scatter it often, so that the winged ones love to come to your wheel. It's also a good idea to put out some food for the slugs and the bugs, for the crawlies and the wigglies to eat, like cornmeal or little pieces of popcorn. Also bring things that they can use to make their homes. When you cut your hair, it's always a good thing to save it and take it to the wheel, leaving it there for the small four-leggeds—like mice—to use to build their houses. The wheel is a place of nurture, and often when you go to it, gifts will be there for you. A winged one will have left you a feather, for example. Skulls and carcasses, skin and feathers are the greatest offerings that those in the animal kingdom can make to us. This is not gross or bad: it is a good thing.

The blessings of the medicine wheel are now yours. The Mystery School is now open. Remembe that in these studies we are in the South, in the south part of the wheel, and that we have entered into the emotional section where we study the seven primary emotions. We are now walking into the space of trust and innocence and growth, honoring the great coyote and its teachings. There will be *heyoka* medicine—that which walks counterclockwise, things that catch you off guard, things that trick you, things that open the door to green. Green is your growth, your beauty, change, and perfection. It is a space where you learn to stand and sing. There you sing your honesty. It is a space that brings about the lessons of faith, of account, of action, and of commitment. Within green you have the opportunity to listen to many words. You have four lessons; you have four medicines; you have a direction; and you have a song. This allows you to have an intimate relationship with the south part of the wheel.

Remember that when you are using a medicine wheel, there is nothing else. The Rainbow Medicine Wheel opens up to every word there is. It also opens you up to every *world* there is. It allows you to sit with the animal kingdom, the plant kingdom, the human kingdom, and the spirit kingdom. It is a place where you can honor Christ, if you want, because there is a cross—the center section represents the red road and the spirit road. But, there is no religion, no doctrine, no creed; nobody is left out of the beauty of the medicine wheel. Take a deep breath in and breathe out. Learn the lessons and allow yourself to live within those things. Walk guilt free, walk disconnected from others, and walk in wholeness in your self.

Aho.

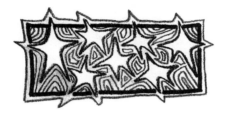

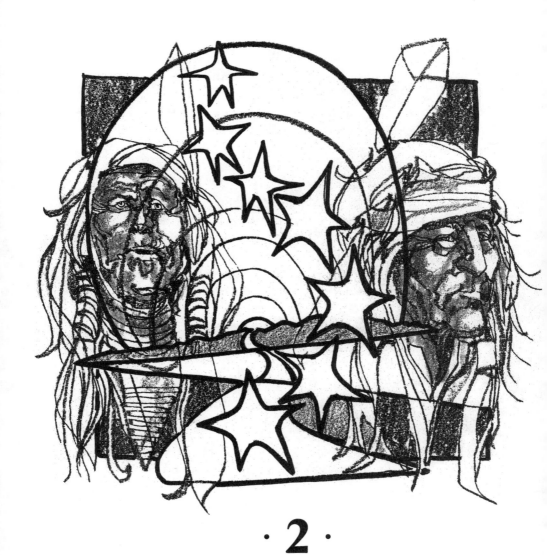

· 2 ·

FACING THE COYOTE—
THE SOUTH

I breathe in and out, and I relax. I feel the earth beneath my feet and the presence of seven with me. I turn and see them. I see their eyes; I see their faces. We sit in a circle in a clearing. There is green grass all around and beautiful stones. Each one of us takes out a rattle and shakes it. We listen to the wind and to the rattles, the sounds softly swaying and gentle. I give my rattle four solid shakes and bring the rattling to an end. There are questions around the circle. "Would you all like to ask them?"

One says to me, "Will I have to give up my Christian ways to study Rainbow Medicine?" Another one says to me, "I'm not sure I want to follow this because it is very strange and unusual." One says, "This is what I have been looking for. I am at home here in nature." One starts crying and has nothing but tears to offer the earth. One looks at me, makes a fist, puts it in the air and pulls it down to her side and says, "YES!" I look at the beauty in these seven people who have chosen to study Star Medicine.

"I look at you and I see you excited about the Dance, the Dance of the Rainbow Self. What I have to offer you is a trip within the spirit world where you are now," and I shake my rattle gently, and watch their fascination. I remember when I came to this. I remember when I stepped into the belief. I thought it was something separate from everything else. I thought that it was a religion of its own. And I remember the gentle old spirit who walked up to me and said, "Darlin', this is no separation. There is no way to separate truth from life. The medicine wheel is ancient. The mystery school is very old. The Teaching Lodge is very beautiful. There is no religion in the medicine wheel, for it is all religion—there is Confidence, Truth, Balance, Creativity, Growth, Wisdom, and Impeccability. There is honor and dishonor alike. There are all the un-words. There are all the emotions here."

My memory of him comes to life, and as I look at that gentle old soul, he begins to dance. He dances around and around and around. His circle gets bigger. He is dancing around us now.

"We must follow him. Listen to his words. He will teach you how to understand. He will show you. He has shown me." I turn, look at him sternly, and say, "Be careful, though, for he is the King, and he knows of what he speaks. He is the guardian of the South. He is the one who holds within him playfulness and trickery. He holds trust and innocence. He is the King of Growth and you must be careful."

I hear a drum, beating slowly, and then faster. "Follow me, and we will go to meet him, see him. Breathe in and out. Look very carefully. Think of the things that you intend to do. Think your intentions very clearly and very carefully."

I look beside the pine tree and there he stands. He is a youth, a young animal, not fully grown. Suddenly—before my eyes—he is in his prime, handsome, powerful. His eyes twinkle in the darkness. His human face is flawless, golden and dark. His animal face is that of a coyote. His fur is strong, rough, and rugged. His nails are able to dig into the earth. He can cling or move fast. He is swift.

"Good noon," he says.

He raises his right hand and in it he has a beautiful green bandanna. He waves it back and forth, left and right. "Let us begin, students. Let the Dance begin, let the games start. Ho, ho, ho, ho, ho," he laughs in a deep, rumbling voice. The drum beats fast and he dances around us, swishing his tail back and forth.

I'm standing in the south gate, looking across at the north. He stops and looks at me. "Aren't you the Wolf? Don't I recognize you?"

I look at him and say, "Yes, King Coyote, but I believe you're standing in my gate."

"Well, I believe you're standing in mine. How does it feel to take on the emotions?"

As I watch him, he ages to become an elderly coyote. Standing in the North, he is in the place of the elder. He grows in wisdom and in his eyes I see a depth. I see lessons of Clarity staring at me face-on.

"There is only one way to achieve your Poise, and that's through me," he says. "It will be through your dance in the fire of your emotions that you will reach the level of Acceptance."

"It would be through my own self that I would reach the level of Acceptance," I said, looking into the fire. "I don't need you. I own my own emotions. I have my own feelings. You simply give me lessons—of heartache."

"It doesn't matter if you own your own emotions. I am emotions, and you'll learn them through me."

"I guess I don't see you as a part of me. I see you as across from me. Emotions are experiences, and you're simply a part of mine."

"Ha, I came, I did, I went—poor poor baby." King Coyote swishes his tail, hunches his back, and bounces around the fire.

I can feel my face turning red. I feel as if my ears are going to explode. "You're ugly," I said, "and you're disgusting!"

He smirks and says, "I am—I'm ugly and I'm disgusting. And not all of us can be a righteous, pious bitch like you. Do you understand what you are?"

"Yes—I'm a white wolf. From the North. Wisdom. A teacher."

"Wouldn't it be interesting to have a wolf trying to teach the emotions," he snarls.

"Are we going to fight every inch of the way?"

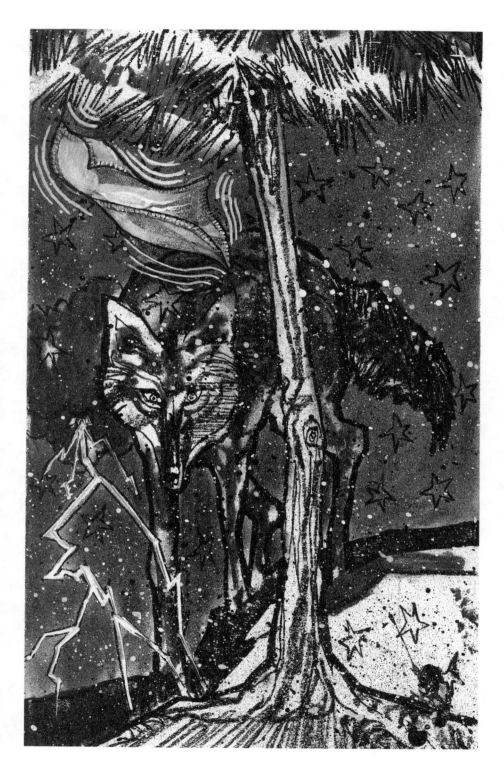

"Well, yes, I would imagine so, if I'm standing in the South and you're standing in the North."

He moves through the air very quickly, a shimmering green glitter all around him. He circles me. He is standing in the South now, looking at me. "Discipline. That will be a lesson that will get you. It will be hard to get up four times a day. I want to see you get up before the crack of dawn every morning and sing the morning star. I want to see you be there at noon and sing the noon sun. I want to see you as the sun sets in the evening, singing the sunset. I want to see you there at midnight, singing the night out." He laughs and says, "I'll watch. I'll watch your discipline. We'll see."

"I take that challenge, King Coyote. I take that challenge and I guarantee you that I have my vision in my heart and I know what I want—"

"Ssh. Bah. Bah. You don't know your vision. You don't even have the ability to have a vision. That's been done away with. Heh, heh, heh," he laughs. "It's been so easy to watch mankind fall away, for there is no discipline. There's simply a feeble attempt at worship."

"I have no doubt. I have no fear, no anger, no sadness that will keep me from living my vision—"

"Like I said, you don't have a vision because you don't know how," the coyote says. "Let me show you what I see."

I feel my eyes getting heavy and I drift off into his mind. I see traffic jams, I see rush hour in the morning. I see gridlock. I see alcohol and drugs, I see broken homes. I see tears and hate. I see people throwing things at each other, pushing and pulling their children. Court cases, bad government. Of course, I see what life is today. I see the quietness of past centuries, the youthfulness of a land 2,000 years ago—gone. Into chaos. I see fire burning homes, buildings being bombed, children being killed.

I hear his laughter. "You want to blame me?" he says. "You want to blame people's emotions. Everything is blame, blame, blame."

Softly the wind blows, and I see his green bandanna take to the air. Way up high the wind takes it, like a kite. It spirals around and around, circles down and quietly drapes itself over a pole. "Here, sit with your emotions. Sit with them like a rock, and learn to grow up. Don't be so whiny. That's called Account. You see, I've shown you things now. I can show you even sadder things."

He begins to dance around the pole. The flute music twinkles underneath his feet. "I can show you many things. I can account for beauty and ugly. I can account for seeing and not seeing. I can account for being successful and unsuccessful. I can account for being weak and being strong. I can account for healing and sickness. I can account for weakness and power. Most of all, I can account for being less than and I can account for great."

He spins, turns, and stops dancing. He looks at me and says, "Long ago, there were seven sacred herbs; there were seven plants that gave their song to the Earth. There was the beauty and healing of the sage, of the sweet grass, of the piñon, of the cedar, the juniper, the osha root, the bitter root. There came forth new herbs from the plant kingdom. They danced their way onto the Earth and sang their songs. They brought you the fact of life. They populated the Earth. And beneath them, life was born. It spiraled about and danced on the Earth, and there was a quietness and a beauty. This was known as the Beauty Way.

"Before the buffalo there was the long yellow grass. Then the buffalo came and it was known as the buffalo grass. Names come to those that stand in the herb and plant kingdom. They know each other as pine and cottonwood. They know each other as seed and flower. They know each other as leaves and needles. They know each other as the natural, magical kingdom of herbs and plants. They know each other as the standing people—they sway and bend with the wind. They were here long before Grandfather, Grandmother brought us here to intermingle and interweave, and live amongst them. They are our teachers. They teach us the healing ways, the way of protection. They give us a knowing. They give us a place to sleep when we gather up their needles and make our beds. They give us healing in the sweet grass, sweet smells that balance the energy, that reduce the anxiety and the fears. They clean and sooth.

"I remember the sage, the pungent aroma in the leaves, that brings about honor—refreshing and balancing the spirit and clearing the mind. I remember the piñon, its strength that some of us nibbled on. We ate from it and it gave us protection and welcomed the spirit in each of us. There was so much brought to the Earth from the sacred—the cedar, the sandalwood, the juniper, the corn. There is so much that comes from the seven sacred herbs. They go on, seven more, to seven more, to seven more, to seven more. And they walk on."

I hear the drum beating softly. I hear the rattle clicking and jingling. King Coyote rubs his face with his paw hand, and shields his left eye, staring down at me out of his right. "What happened to the Beauty Way, Wolf? Where did such ugliness come from? Shall we blame *my* direction? Shall we say it's all the emotions' fault?"

"Well, Coyote, you do hold people captive. Emotions have driven people crazy."

"It is not emotions that do that, Wolf. It is the entwining, entangling, pulling, and rushing. It is forces beyond the emotions that cause the devastation. Pushing and pulling, twisting and turning, crossing. These are not emotions. These are forces."

In front of me is a pole with a green flag attached. I find myself sitting cross-legged, looking at it. "I *do* want to blame my emotions. I want to get mad and say it is the madness itself that makes things even worse."

He sits next to me, his back next to mine, King Coyote, my emotions themselves. "The trickery is only in the push and pull. The tension, the anxiety, the madness is force itself. Emotions are necessary. You don't want to get rid of your Acceptance. You don't want to get rid of your fear. Pick an emotion that you would want to get rid of. Oh, Wolf, you know that the Dance of the South, the Rainbow Self, is all about how you feel. You've been there before, and you'll go there again. And you always seem to want me to be the reason. Blame the emotions."

"Yeah, I'll blame you, Coyote, I will blame the emotions. It's emotions that keep me out of balance."

In spite of myself I'm enjoying sitting there swaying in the breeze with my back against his. It's familiar and comfortable, but I don't trust him.

"Yeah, yeah, yeah, it's about trust, Wolf. See how easy it is to let go of your trust and start to blame? It's easy to blame—blame your anger, blame your fear, blame your sadness—blame it all. But your joy is affected. I know you're not happy. Basically, the best thing to do to draw on your strength is to sit still and accept. Gather up your Acceptance. It is the way it is. Yeah, you might have a long, hard pull from there."

"Well, I do. I listen to students who have been lied to and stolen from," I say, "molested and raped—"

He jumps up and stands in front of me in all his ferocity, teeth showing. He says, "They'll just have to accept it! I can't say it any clearer!"

Oh, there goes that lightning and here goes the thunder, and the South and the North begin to clash. He takes a deep breath and looks at me. He says, "I may be just a little scrawnier than you, 'cause a wolf is a little bigger than a coyote, but we certainly are relatives." He pauses. "You can't pull the North and South apart. You can't tear them apart. You can't take the thunder and lightning and separate them and have a storm. You can't take the mind and the emotions apart. What do you know about the mind, Wolf?"

"I stand in the mind. I *am* the mind. I'm from the North. The teachings of Grandfather, Grandmother Wolf are the teachings of the mind. It is the soul, the hallway to the stars."

"Ah! The stars." Coyote smiles. "The stars! Watch the stars," and he holds out his hand. As he does, the thunder rolls and stars drip from his fingertips. At first they are a beautiful blue; then they are green; then they are purple. As they hit the ground, they bounce and scatter in reds and oranges, yellows and burgundies; then there are greens and purples, and they intermingle, twist, turn, and scatter to the edges of the earth.

"Ah. The South. The emotions. The dance. Star Medicine. Let us calm the storm and stop the fight between lightning and thunder. Let us be at peace on the physical road."

I see the sincerity in his eyes. Maybe the Coyote isn't such a bad old guy after all. I turn to the North, and there he is again, as an Elder. I see him as one who has taught his heart out. Now he walks with a limp and a cane. I see him as the grandest. He is my feelings. He is my reason for living. Without a mind, there are no feelings. Without feelings there is no mind.

"Maybe this Acceptance is not so bad after all, Coyote."

He laughs. He is in the center—now a man, a coyote dancer. There he stands—innocent and clear, strength and success. "It's yours. It's yours to teach them, Wolf. Don't let them forget the beauty. Bring it to life in the flowers. Give them a dozen roses. Teach them not to stop smelling the beauty. Open their doors to balance their emotions. Take them into the noon sunshine. But I'll bet you that within 72 hours after they have heard you speak, they'll forget. And you'll feel disgust, 'cause that's human nature.

"Let me tell you something, Wolf. Take the message back to Earth, to the two-legged, that they need to walk gently on each other. Because they are going to be elders, and then they're going to be older, and then they're going to be elderly, and then they're going to be ancestors. Then it's going to be too late to do anything about it. Will they have grasped the storm between you and me? Will they understand the thunder and the lightning?"

His eyes dim to a dark green. He turns into a pine tree in front of my face. The wind blows him up to four hundred feet—a huge grandfather pine tree swaying in the wind. I have never seen such a grand sight, such a large pine!

I sit there and the rain comes through the pine needles and drips around me. I pull down my black hat and prepare to teach. I know that what lies ahead of me could only be one thing, and that is a solid, gentle hallway within the soul. For the storm becomes soft and the Dance of the Rainbow Self comes forth as we sit right here in this circle and play the drum softly. I cannot promise you that life will be easy. I cannot wave a magic wand over everything and make it all right. But I can say that when you take a deep breath in, and let it out, and step outside of yourself into your spirit— emotions don't seem so bad after all, if you can look at them through

Acceptance. I know these words to be true, but they are my words; they are my walk.

I hear the soft sounds of the stars calling me back.

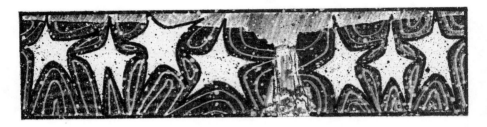

The Pole with the Green Flag

Tools: *A 7-foot (2m) pole, a piece of green cloth 3 inches (7.5cm) wide by 36 inches (1m) long; 17 rocks; a shovel for digging a hole; smudging tools; a white candle. If you're doing the ceremony indoors, stand the pole on the floor and prop it up with rocks, in a room tall enough to have a 7-foot pole in it.*

The seventeen rocks should be six to ten inches (15 to 25cm) across. Seven of the rocks are Medicine Words, which are Strength, Success, Vision, Beauty, Healing, Power, and Great. Seven of the rocks are Lesson Words, which are Clarity, Poise, Discipline, Account, Fact, Sense, and Complete. One rock is for Trust, one rock is for Innocence, and one is for Growth.

Select a quiet place where you will be undisturbed. If it is indoors, it should be a room with nothing in it. Remove all the furniture and clear the room out totally. It will be a place where you go to sit and listen to Trust, Innocence, and Growth.

Dig a hole, place the seven-foot pole solidly in the ground, and tie the green cloth around the pole. Then place the rocks around the bottom of the hole to hold the pole securely. First, place the Medicine Rock of Strength along with the Lesson Rock of Clarity. To have Strength you must learn to be clear.

Sit with your spirit journal and ask yourself this question: "What keeps me from having my clarity?" Next, place the Medicine Rock of Success along with the Lesson Rock of Poise. Again ask yourself, "What keeps me from having my Success? What takes away my Poise?" When you have journaled that answer, move on to the next rock, the Vision rock. Place it along with the Lesson Rock of Discipline. Ask yourself, "What keeps me from having my medicine of Vision? What keeps me from doing my Disciplines?" Then place the rock of Beauty, along with the Lesson Rock of Account, and ask yourself, "What keeps me from having my Beauty? What keeps me from Account?" Next, place the rock of Healing, the lesson of Fact. Ask, "What keeps me from Healing? What keeps me from Fact?" Journal your answers. Then place the rock of Power and the Lesson Rock of Sense, and asks, "What keeps me from having my Power? What keeps me from Sense?" Answer those questions in your journal. Then place the rock of Great and the Lesson Rock of Complete. Ask yourself, "What keeps me from being Great? What keeps me from being Complete?"

If you answer your questions, "Nothing. I am those things," your words will make the flag move. Then you honor them by standing up and actually blowing the flag. If you want, you can wave your hand back and forth to create a breeze, or use a fan to move the flag.

Intention Ceremony

Your intention is vital to your Success, and the ceremony of Intention helps you to form your purpose, goal, or aim, or to focus on the object you wish, your vision or your dream. It gives it greater meaning and helps you to plan and make decisions. If you have things that keep you from your medicines or you have things that you have not learned within your Lesson Words, it is now time to set the intentions. At your green flag pole, you set your Intention Ceremony in motion by

1. **Making a commitment to yourself.** I want to learn how to be strong—I want my Strength. I want to have Success. I want my Vision. I want my Beauty. I want a Healing. I want Power, I want to be Great. I will learn the lesson of Clarity. I will have my Poise. I will do my Discipline. I will Account for things. I will know the Facts. I will have the Facts. I will make Sense, and I will be Complete.

2. **Setting your intentions** by typing a prayer for each one of these, in the color that it is—Strength and Clarity in red, Success and Poise in orange, Vision and Discipline in yellow, Beauty and Account in Green, Healing

and Fact in blue, Power and Sense in purple, and Great and Complete in burgundy.

3. Tying those prayers to the Pole. When you do this you are making a commitment to have those things. Once you have tied the prayers to the pole, sit down and write out what they are for you.

> *Example: My Strength is knowing my Vision, finding my Vision at a young age. My Success is living my Vision, teaching, bringing forth a teaching career. Not bending to anyone's description of what I should be. My Vision is the sun, the moon, and the seven stars, and I know my Vision and I listen to it. My Beauty is knowing that I have my Strength. I can see it in my walk. I look in the mirror and see the green in my eyes and I know that I have my Beauty. Healing: Any time my weakness comes, I turn to my teachings and I know I have my Strength. Power. Looking at others who have taken on Rainbow Medicine, have listened to their Vision, have remembered their ancestry, and have found their belief. Great: A feeling I have as I sit here and write.*

4. Lighting a white candle at the base of the green flag pole. Do that once a day, every day, to make a commitment to this ceremony.

If you are in an area where you cannot get a pole or have a piece of ground, you can do the ceremony as a visual exercise. Simply sit very quietly in your chair, close your eyes, and see each thing that I have said in your mind's eye, and let your spirit walk on the earth. Let your mind, your emotions, and your spirit become total. Let go of your physicality. When you do these ceremonies in your mind, you are actually doing them in your spirit. So visualize each thing very clearly, and do it. Bring it back and write about it in your journal. Be sure to use the journal, though, for a physical connection. There is no place where you can't have a journal.

It is very important to set an intention for the south part of the wheel, which is Star Medicine. You need to know what you want to achieve from your emotions, what you want to learn from your emotions, what you want to remember from your emotions, and how you want to deal with your emotions—for your primary emotions are the basic stairways to the rest of your existence. This is especially true in Success, because Success is achieved through your Acceptance, your Happiness and your Joy. You need to achieve Balance in your Anger, in your Fear, and in your Sadness. You must understand the things that Disgust you and cause you to push away, to knock down, to tear down. These things are movements of your emotions that get in the way of your Success. For you to have your Poise, to learn the lesson of Poise, is to regain your Strength. You do that by setting a Balance in your Success. And doing that, you need to look inside yourself and come to Acceptance of the way things are.

In an intention ceremony, it is good to ask yourself the question "Why did I do what I did?" and find the answer. Once you have found that answer, move on to what you are going to do now. "What will I take from what I did and how will I use it in my walk today?" It doesn't matter whether you are limited to four walls or chained; it doesn't matter if you are bound in a bad relationship; there is always a way to move on in Greatness. Great is the word that opens the door so that you can step out into your fullness. When you want to reach your fullness, it is possible to get Greatness from every moment you have. There should be no whining, no bitterness, and your sadness should be Balanced, because you are able to learn from everything you do. You take all the lessons and they are the lessons of Clarity. You put them in motion and they become teachings.

Through our intentions, we turn our lessons into something solid. That means that we understand Clarity and through our Clarity we understand Poise. Through our Poise we understand Disciplines. In our Disciplines in life, we Account. This brings us into a place where intentions are Fact. Everything is very solid and very clear. That Fact makes Sense, and we move on into Complete. When that happens, we've walked the road of the lessons in the South in our emotions. Set your Intention Ceremony to open yourself to those things.

Ceremony of Trust

Tools: *Cornmeal; your spirit journal and pen; a white votive candle in a holder; a green cloth; yarn or string. You will also need forty leaves. They can be new or old leaves, or they can be leaves cut out of paper. You'll need access to a fire for burning the leaves or a river to let them float down. Once again, if you don't have the opportunity to get outdoors to do these things, you can do them in your mind and think about going to a river or going to a fire when needed.*

1. **Preparation of the ceremony of trust.** Place your green cloth on the ground. Set a white candle in a holder in the center. Have your journal and pen nearby. Make a cornmeal circle all around yourself, so you are sitting

in the middle, encompassed with Growth and goodness and Nurture, which is what the cornmeal stands for.

2. Sit and list in your journal what you trust and what you don't trust.

3. Question and list: What do the things that you trust have to do with?

Example: I trust my boss. It has to do with my job.

List all your trusts and what they have to do with. Then write each one on a piece of paper, place it on a leaf and tie it onto the leaf; or you can write it onto the leaf itself. If necessary you can simply place it onto the leaf, in your mind's eye, or think it onto the leaf.

4. Next, make a list of things you don't trust, and place them on the leaves.

5. Sit with the things that you don't trust, and understand your "don't trusts." The how's, the why's, the what's. When you are working on regaining Trust, the most important thing is to answer what happened—to get to what we call the core—to find out why it happened. Answer them with the medicines.

Example: I was weak and let my Strength down, therefore I did not believe in myself and I lost my job. I was unSuccessful because I didn't know how to do better. I allowed myself to be a failure. I couldn't see—I had no Vision. I had nothing to help me or guide me. I had no teachings, I had no answers, and therefore I struck out in Anger. I wanted to be ugly, full of darkness and hate, bitter, and evil. I rejected Beauty and therefore I have nobody in my life. I am ill and I need help. I need a Healing. I have no cure; no solidity. Therefore, I am sick and I am dying. I have no self. I am weak, my self-esteem is low, therefore I have no Power. When I have no Power, I cannot achieve. I have no Greatness. I don't see myself as anything except worthless, so therefore that's what I am.

When you look through your negatives, look at the negative sides of the words. Draw in the self-pity and see what you are doing to yourself. Is it yours not to see? Is it yours not to want? Is it yours not to be? Is it yours not to have? As you sit with the leaves and you start to understand the depth of your negativity, begin to be excited about your Strength. *I can!* Find something in your mind that you have accomplished and bring it forth as a Strength—something good that you did in your life. Then bring a Success into your mind. Bring something that you did that was successful—see it happening. Bring something that is Beautiful to your mind. Bring in a Healing that happened. Bring Power into your life, as you brought Completeness and Success into your experience. And bring Greatness into your life—even if it's nothing more than one moment when you blew out a birthday candle; it was your moment.

It is important, as you let go of your lack of trust on the leaves, that you bring the medicines into your self and bring Trust into Balance. Trust is a part of the South that allows you to come forth in the fullness of your emotions. You cannot always sit in negatives and dwell on them. That would get you nowhere. You must bring forth the good and build the habit of Success, the habit of Confidence within Strength, the habit of Vision—so that you are able to look forward to your Vision and make Sense. Let it be a platform beneath you—a personal experience with a Healing, a personal experience with your Beauty. When you are working with these things, and are sure that you have them all intact, place the things that you do not trust in the fire and let them burn away. Or put them on the water and let them float away. Or, bury them and forget them.

Breathe in, and remember the Strengths. Take the things that you do trust, that you have written on the leaves, and throw them in the air. Let them float down around you and scatter. Then stand on them. Your Trust is now solid. Journal it. Keep it. Look at the leaf you stand on. Look at the one that falls on your head. Look at the leaf that lands on your foot, look at the one you've got to walk on. And understand where you are going. Your Trust should be your medicine. I trust my Strength. I see the Strength in myself. I trust Greatness. I strive to be Great. I do not give my Power to anything but myself, for I draw on my Power to be as Powerful as I can be. Then I will walk in my Greatness. My Greatness is my Trust.

Ceremony of Innocence

Tools: *Two dozen and seven sticks. The sticks need to be 10 to 15 inches (25–37cm) long. You'll need 24 inches (60cm) of green cloth cut 3 inches (7.5cm) wide; seven colors of yarn or thread—red, orange, yellow, green, blue, purple, and burgundy; a candle; smudge bowl, herbs, and matches; spirit journal and pen.*

The ceremony of innocence is brought about from the South. It is a good idea to use the pole with the green flag (see pages 51–52), but you may do this ceremony in your mind or use a pole that already exists in a public place.

Tie the strip of cloth to the pole. Light the candle and place it at the base of the pole. Take four deep breaths—in through your nose and out through your mouth. After the fourth breath, relax and let go of what is worrying you. Let go of your busy days, let go of your questions, let go of everything, and just stand there in quiet and peace. Sit on the ground and open your journal.

First you need to establish what innocence is. Most of the time we are taught that innocence has to do with sexuality, but that is just one facet of our lives. Innocence is pure, faultless, safe, childlike, open, simple, and right. One of the spirits of the South is innocence. There is innocence, intention, growth, and trust. When you are working in the south part of the medicine wheel, it is up to you to regain these things or to know that you are stable and balanced in all of them. The ceremony of innocence is meant to re-unite you with your pure, with your faultless, with your right, with your safe, with your childlike, your open, and your simple.

Make a list of the loss of your innocence. List where you lost your pure, where you lost your faultless, where you began to have faults, and list those faults. List your wrongs—where you turned away from what you felt was right. List your safe, where you became unsafe. List where you lost our childlike, where you became adult and hardened. List the loss of your open, where you became closed. List the loss of your simple, where you became complicated.

> *Example: Looking forward to Christmas and feeling joy and anticipation was lost by understanding that there was no Santa Claus—no one who would make your life better, no magic that would make what you wanted appear under a Christmas tree.*

When you have these in mind and are solid with all the losses of your innocence, take a stick. You have seven sticks for the regaining of your innocence, and two dozen sticks to use for your losses. If you have more losses than the two dozen sticks, gather others. Write on a piece of paper each loss of innocence that you have, wrap it around the stick, and tie it with a red cord, for you are seeking the red path, the Red Road. You are wanting to regain your Strength and stand in the fullness of your spirit.

When you have listed all of your losses of innocence and tied them onto sticks, sit with the sticks and think about the anger that is connected to these losses. Take time in your journal to work through why they have happened. Be honest with yourself. Be truthful. Write down what you have walked away from and what you have turned away from. Keep this knowledge in your journal so that you remember where you have turned your back on your innocence and where your innocence has been lost. Look at these pages in your journal often.

When you have completed the losses of your innocence, take control by breaking the sticks. Break them in half and put them in a pile. When you have broken all the sticks, look at the pile.

Now take the seven sticks that are left. Wrap the first one with red string or yarn, knowing that it is your Strength. Think about how you will regain your pure through your Strength—pure being clean and clear, fresh and new. Think of regaining that through Strength.

> **Example:** *You have a problem saying no when you need to. No is a pure answer and very helpful. "Do you drink alcohol?" You don't—but you don't say no because maybe the person asking is a drinker and wants you to drink and won't care about you if you don't say yes. So, you don't want to say no, but you have put your red string on the stick and you say, "No, I don't drink." It is your pure answer because it is your belief and you want and need to say no. Then the person says, "Well, I like to drink and have people around me who drink." You are then very clean and clear. "I don't drink," and "No, I am not going to drink alcohol, and if I need to leave, I will." The person says, "I need you to go because we don't need someone who will ruin our fun." So you walk. Your fresh and new response comes alive because always before you would bend and do what someone else wanted you to do. Think of your newfound strength, and hold this pure, clean, clear, fresh, and new innocence close to your heart.*

With the second stick, think of your faults and what they have been. Think of how you will win over your faults by becoming successful. How you will stand strong in your Success and overcome your faults. You will replace your faults by undoing them and turning them into Proper, into Successes. Wrap your stick with orange.

Think of your wrongs and how you wish to turn them into right. With the third stick, see yourself becoming right and doing the things that you want to do. Make a list of things that you would like to have come for you— for example, freedom, happiness, marriage, success, strength—and see those things. See yourself being happy. Get a mental picture of yourself standing in the sunshine. Draw a breath in and out, and relax. Understand that your rights are coming into their fullness by your Vision. Wrap this stick with yellow.

Wrap the next stick in green. See the things that are unsafe for you, the things that you wish to make safe. Achieve them by putting the medicine Beauty to work. Bring as much Beauty into your life as you can. Think of the right things to do through reaching out to Beauty, obtaining your Safe.

> *Example: To feel safe is to know—knowing there is no hate, anger, or rage. These actions are shown in daily life by hateful angry words, name-calling, fighting, guns, shooting at each other. All of these actions cause a person to feel unsafe. Beauty, which is found in color, nature, strength—and examples of strength in others—is what treats a lot of unsafe actions. When we see the beauty of sharing and the look of love in others' eyes, we get a safe feeling. Beauty can also be doing things correctly and having things clear. Also it can be Clarity within our homelife—taking care of the home, taking care of money matters, children, and animals—all of this is Beauty.*

Wrap the next stick in blue. See the things that are gone from your childlike, the things that have broken the child within you and turned it cold and hard, things that have made you grow up, made you solid in being cold. See a Healing, a transformation that brings about a new playfulness, that gives zest and vigor, the ability to anticipate. Bring back your childlike by applying the medicine of Healing.

> *Example: Christmas is the time of the child, birthday also—going to the park or the zoo—playing with other children or a family pet. All of these are examples of childlike. You have no use for any of them. You have bad memories of Christmas, never celebrated birthdays, never have been allowed to play or go to the park or the zoo, never have had a pet or children. But now you have friends who have children, and you have the chance to see Christmas in a new light. Their birthdays are a time you want to make special. "Special" is the magic. You set out to care, and that is the zest and vigor. Now you are grown, you have work, yourself, and freedom to give to others. You show those who are little now how important ceremony and celebration are by having simple holidays and honoring their birthdays. You are in the childlike when life is simple.*

To work with the open, wrap the next stick in purple, the Power medicine.

Power allows you to flow. Look at the things that have caused you to be closed and shut down, things that have taken away your openness. List your most powerful thoughts and your most powerful attributes, the things that make you who you are. When you look within your Power, you balance your flow and it gives you the ability to have what you can see. When you put your Power medicine to work, you realize what you can achieve, not what someone else can do for you or what someone else can make you be, but what *you* can do.

> *Example: Power within human life is Strength, the ability to believe, to have faith. Often it is the church or spiritual teachings that supply our Power. Having a good job and being able to support yourself and your family gives you self-esteem. Self-esteem in general is Power. Good health, and having an education and skills, is Power. To study and know what you are able to do is Power. Gifts of tradition, the name of a family, belonging and fitting in are Power. Gifts of the Spirit, a vision, a calling to the message of God is Power. I find that knowing, safety, fairness, and richness of spirit are the most powerful.*

Next is your burgundy, your simple. Simple is restored with Great medicine. Great is uplifting. It is giant and expansive. It seems hard to equate that with simple but simple is vast and complex. It becomes simple in the fact that it is. So to restore your simple in life, go to what just "is" for you.

Often we confuse "is" with addictions. We look at cravings and obsessions as what is. "What is" is what is normal for you. It would be your family's tradition; it would be your hereditary choices; it would be what is natural for you, what you like—that is natural. What "is" is never an outside substance. It is always an inside feeling. You draw your "is" from your simple, and your simple comes from your open. Which comes from your childlike, your child heart. Your child heart is a song your spirit sings. To obtain Great for you, you have to look inside the pure of your thoughts to find your song, and bring your thoughts into their fullness. Thoughts have no faults and they have no wrongs. Thoughts are pure and simple. Through simple, pure thought we obtain Great. Great medicine is Greatness. A great mind is strong and pure. It brings about a witness, through your actions, of Strength and Success. There you will see your Beauty. A movement is at hand.

> *Example: A person sits and thinks, listens to the elders, looks at the mistakes others make and also the power, correctness, and good that others*

do, the helping, caring, and feeling good about self that can be seen in others. Then the person sets out a plan, makes up lists, sets goals for action in these good ways. The person studies teachers, listens to wise experience, and puts all of this behavior in motion—doing what is learned from teachers, elders, wise ones, and bringing it forth in life, having students themselves. One grows from this correct, good, powerful teaching, and others' lives bring Great to its fullness. The cycle of life is seen through Great—mom, daughter, granddaughter, father, son, grandson— teacher-student.

Look back at the seven sticks that you have wrapped with the seven colors and be grateful for them. Look at your red and write down how it feels to have your Strength. List your strengths.

: my beauty, my intelligence, my kindess.

ır orange, and list your Successes.

: knowing myself, being able to know others, being able to be

ır yellow and list your Vision.

Example: *the sun, the moon, and the seven stars: The sun being able to have direction, the stars being able to lay out a path, and the moon being able to celebrate the totality of that path.*

Look at your green and see your Beauty.

Example: *the way I can see my Vision, the way I write my Vision to enable others, the way I believe in my Vision.*

Look at your blue and see your Healing.

Example: *I could have been something else—spending my time in a job behind a computer or raising children—but I have kept my heart connected to the Beauty Way and to the Path and now I teach shamanism and the Rainbow Path.*

Look at the purple and see your Power.

61

Example: the opportunity to teach the south part of the wheel and to show what my emotions are, to speak forth primary emotions and give directions on how to understand philosphies of life. I have within me the Power of knowledge from my colors.

Look at the burgundy and see your Greatness and list that.

Example: the mail I receive from students about my book, the students who draw strength from me and enjoy their lives from their studies and the teachings they follow.

You have the opportunity now to look at your Ceremony of Innocence and see that you have restored your pureness, that you are faultless, that your rights are solid, that you are safe, that you're childlike, open, and simple. Keep working on this ceremony until you feel all of this in motion for you. When you have these things, continue through life with a fullness and a richness. Understand that you have been in the presence of the south gate, and that you have been face to face with the coyote. You have looked at your emotions and have applied your medicines from the South. Now you have the opportunity to go on to the lessons that lie ahead in this book on the South.

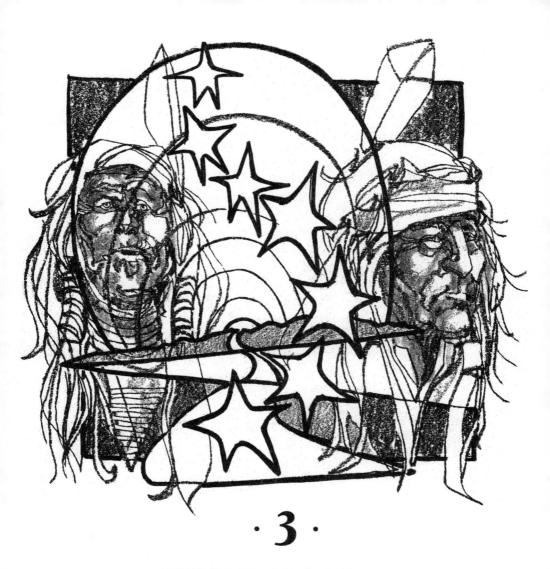

· 3 ·

THE DANCE OF
THE RED ROSE

I walk to the east gate. I enter, raising my hands to the sky, taking a deep breath, and spinning around clockwise as I step into the wheel. I am standing in the spirit. I move clockwise, passing each medicine of the spirit. I face South. Lifting my hands to the air, I give thanks and honor to Great Spirit. I draw in four deep breaths and relax.

I am walking along a path. This path is in a well-manicured garden, a park setting in which the grass is perfect. Before me I see a flower bed with beautiful roses. I see a park bench where I sit and look at the blue sky. I breathe in and out, and I relax. I feel sadness in my heart. I am weakened; I am destroyed. I am sad; I am empty; I feel alone. I feel tears start to run down my face. I feel the wind circle around me four times. I smell the exquisite fragrance of roses. I continue to cry and to breathe.

The park has become a forest and I am deep within it. In front of me there is a magnificent red rose bush, single and alone.

"Get up, young one," I hear. "Go and circle the rose bush four times. Draw from it its Beauty. Draw from it its Strength. Receive a Healing from it and regain your Power. Feel this and have your Success. Take a deep breath and smell the rose in all its Greatness."

The voice is deep and solid, rich and full. The rose bush is exceptionally lovely. Its leaves are rich and a lustrous green; its buds are two thumbs thick. The blossoms are as big around as a teacup and not fully opened yet. Deep and rich red, they are.

I rise and circle the rose bush four times, as I was told. As I do, the air around me turns a soft red—the sky, the air—everything is a very soft red. The wind blows softly through the pines that surround me. The grass is rich and green, with pine needles scattered around. I sit on a bench and from the rose bush a dancer appears. There is the sound of a drum and a flute. The dancer takes a prancing step and marches to the tune of the drum and the flute. The sky begins to shimmer with red stars—twinkling spots of light. The dancer circles the rose bush, prancing and raising his knees, stepping and marching. He carries two rattles in each hand. The rattles are made of bells and he is shaking them. The rattles twinkle, glisten, and clatter as the spirit dances around the rose bush. The dancer has a full set of elk horns. I see that he is part elk and part man. His legs are painted red with white stripes. He has moccasins on his feet, beaded in red and white. He wears a loincloth made of elk skin with the hair on it in the front. He is bare from the waist up, but he has a cape made of elk skin over his shoulder. His chest is painted red and he has white dots on his back. The left side of his face is elk and the right side of his face is human.

As he dances, he changes. He becomes all elk, and then at times he becomes all man. When he is man, he is beautiful. His features are strong, his eyes intense and dark. His chest is broad and thick, his muscles expanded. I watch him dance around the rose until the sorrow in my heart begins to drift away. He walks up to me and extends his hand. In it he has a fistful of red stars. He throws them into the air and, as he does, rose petals

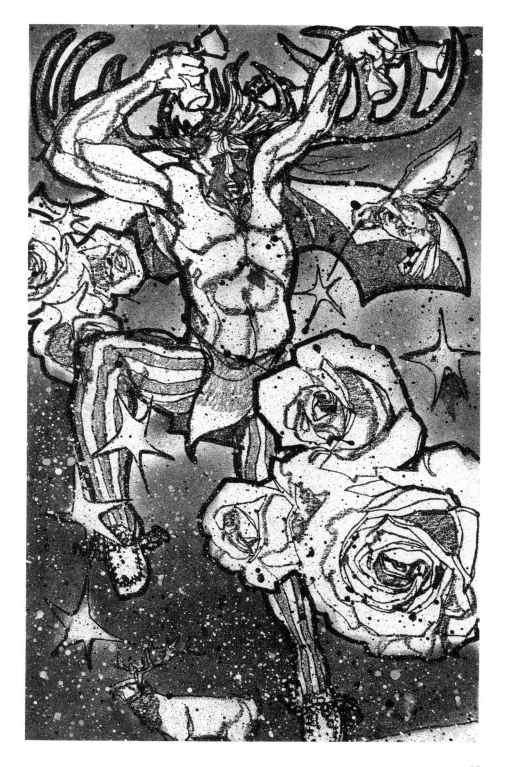

fall all around me—red rose petals cover the ground—hundreds of them fall from the sky. The fragrance is overpowering. He kneels on one knee in front of me, and he says, "I am Water Elk. I am Strength. I am the spirit of the heart of the rose. I am Strength medicine. You must let go. You must remember that sympathy is a feeling of learning. It is a place where you go to honor. You have lost an elder to death. You grieve from the loss. Your heart must be cleaned. You are just a young one in your mind, and it is hard to lose a mom. It is hard to lose an elder who is mom to you."

I hear him, and a drum beating behind him. He moves away quickly, as an animal does through the forest, and there he stands at the edge of the trees, a full mature elk, head turned toward the sky, horns dipped to the right. I hear singing, a Native chant. The drum is still beating softly; the wind is calling me. For I have lost an elder. I remember the greatest pain I have ever felt, the death of a mom. For when I was young on earth I was placed in the hands of a very wise and kind German woman, who raised and guided me. It isn't an unusual thing for a Native mother to let go of her child. In the days when I was young, times were hard and money was scarce and my mother reached out to someone to give me guidance, family, and love. She placed me with her adopted aunt—a beautiful, gentle soul. The greatest pain I have ever borne is the loss of that mom when I was seven—a sadness that ripped my heart from its cage.

I breathe in and out as I look at the elk ahead of me and listen to his song. He bellows in the air. Then, before my eyes he returns as a spirit man.

"Death is a doorway," he says. "It is an opportunity to learn to accept. Acceptance is a balancing you will need in your life to give your Strength its fullness. There are times, Wolf, that each of your students—that each of us on Earth—feels as if our heart has been broken. There is a time when that kind one, that loved one, or perhaps that child, is removed from our presence and we are sad." He holds out his left hand and in it is a hummingbird. He opens his hand and the hummingbird stands on the back of his hand. He says, "Clearly, look. Clarity is in front of you, the lesson. The lesson itself."

I watch the hummingbird lift up off his hand and hover like a helicopter. It flies backwards and darts in front of us. It trembles over the rose bush and then moves beyond. I see very clearly. The lesson of clarity is at hand. I could cry for many moons, year upon year, in sadness and grief over death. Or I could see what I see in front of me.

"Wolf, in front of you is the path of stars. Can you see it?"

There on the ground I see glistening stars—silvers and whites, with hints of red.

"Follow the path. Regain your Strength and hold it in Acceptance."

I begin to walk and feel a force come over me. It is courage. I can look back at my childhood and let go of all my fear now. In front of me I see a boldness. It is a spirit. It is a spirit of all colors. It is a doorway. The doorway has an opening of brightness, the brightest light I have ever seen.

"Intensity, toughness, hardness—these are your choices. As your guide, I ask you to bring them within you now. Breathe them in."

I take a deep breath and smell the oil of the rose. I feel the balancing of the grief in my heart. I let my eyes slowly close. I feel courage inside me. I have only one desire, and that is to follow the path—to have Strength, to build a base, to allow myself the courage and vigor to hold Strength in its fullness.

"Acceptance is a guarantee, Wolf. It's a clarification, an acknowledgment. Here in this land that you see before you there is only a recognition of sadness as a doorway. That doorway where the brightness is, you have now stepped through. Look into the spirit world, Wolf. Find her."

Before me there is a small, simple house with a beautiful flower garden in the front yard. It has a porch, with her familiar fishing chair sitting at the front. A little sign is hung out saying "Baker." I know that it is mom and daddy's house. I walk up the simple rock pathway, jump up on the porch, and knock at the front door. The gentle soul comes to the front door with her apron on, dusted with flour. She has been making an apple pie. She looks at me with her blue eyes and smiles.

"Today's a great day for you," she says, "for you have seen the brightness and you have stepped beyond your sadness. I am always alive."

Behind her I see Daddy Baker put his arms around her. "We're right here, child. Right here, in your Strength, where we've always been."

I return through the brightness. I am standing before the rose bush. I look at the beauty of the rich, red color of the rose. I look into the rose, and there I see a marvelous shirt with symbols painted on it and little ribbons of color hanging from it. The symbols seem familiar. In front of me I see the river—rushing, winding, moving on. It is crystal clear. I look back at the symbols on the shirt.

"Take this shirt home with you, Wolf," Water Elk says. "Remember what it looks like in your mind, and bring it forth. Make it happen because it is your spirit shirt. It is there for you to know, to hold, to open, and to be. The spirit shirt holds the symbols that tell you about each one of your medicines. See that path along the river?"

I look and there is a familiar path.

"Follow it. Dance the Dance of the Red Rose. Follow your spirit symbols.

You will come across the teachings of the Earth, the teachings of the Yellow Bird, and other teachings that open doors for you. There is a lot to learn about your emotions. There are feelings within Sadness and Disgust, feelings within Fear. But you have words to bring back to share with your students. You will allow each one of them to know that during their time on Earth they are given the opportunity to draw from the depth of the medicine, to reach within the spirit world and have the answers. You must remember what you have seen today—that the dear ones you love are alive and well in the spirit world. You must always have faith in that."

"But the separation, Water Elk, it makes me so, so sad. I'm way past seven now and many, many years have passed, but the sadness of them not being there . . ."

"Well, in the physical you have a choice," he says. "Think of the Greatness. Look for the mist, because beyond it is the Great Waterfall. Always keep your mind on the Great Waterfall. There you will find the secrets. You will hold within your heart the knowledge of the emotions. Everything in life isn't given at one moment. You cannot know everything in one moment. But Strength allows you to have the force of the spirit; it gives you courage. You hold it in a boldness, an intensity, and a hardness that builds a base, that opens the brightness, and there you step through in a breath. You have your courage. Strength shall never leave you. Head towards the Waterfall, Wolf."

The stars shimmer above my head and their soft voices call me.

I hear the soft sounds of the stars calling me back.

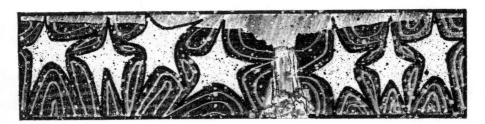

Mini-Wheels

A mini-wheel is a wheel within a wheel, one that allows you to take a specific spot and study it.

Example: You are within the South, and within the South is the teaching of emotions. In a mini-wheel, emotions are in the center, and around the center are the seven primary emotions, which are Acceptance, Disgust, Happy, Sad, Anger, Fear, and Joy. This becomes a mini-wheel of emotions.

To make a mini-wheel, place a stone in the center and four stones in a circle arund the center, as shown in the picture. Then draw the circle in your journal and add the words given here. Apply the words one at a time and write about them in your journal while you work with the wheel in your life. Keep the mini-wheel set up while you work with intention.

The Concept of the Emotion
(Understanding of actions,
Purpose, Strength, Thought)

The Totality of the Emotion
(Seen in physical life,
understandings, fruits,
knowledge, personality)

EMOTION

The Spirit of the Emotion
(Clarity, everlastingness,
illumination, enlightenment)

The Feeling of the Emotion
(Depth, the way you affect,
the way you are affected,
outcome of actions)

Wheels Within Wheels

You can also take each emotion and set it in place as a wheel. Start with Acceptance. Put Acceptance in the center and give it its four directions (see the wheel on page 70). For each emotion, there is the spirit of the emotion, the feelings of the emotion, the totality of the emotion, and the concept of the emotion. The spirit of the emotion is its clarity and its everlastingness, its illumination, and enlightenment. The feelings of the emotion are its depth, the way you are affected, the way you affect, and the outcome of actions that you take from the emotion itself. The totality of the emotion is the way it can be seen in your physical life, the understandings that you have and demonstrate in your physical life, the fruits of your labors that are the attributes and knowledge of the emotion, as well as your basic personality from moment to moment, hour to hour, day to day. The concept of the emotion is the understanding that you base your actions upon. It is your understanding of your purpose, operating from the emotion. It's your inner strength that brings forth your motivation. And it's your mind's thought—the actual thought process that you are experiencing at any given moment.

The Emotional Teachings of Acceptance

On a piece of paper, or using stones or objects, make a mini-wheel for Acceptance. Place Acceptance in the center and on the right-hand side place the spirit. At the bottom place the feelings. To the left-hand side place totality and on top place the concept. In the spirit section, place the word "guarantee." In the feelings section, place the word "belief." In the totality place "clarification." In the concept place "acknowledgment."

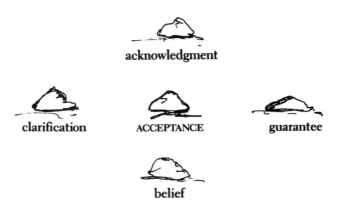

acknowledgment

clarification   ACCEPTANCE   guarantee

belief

In your spirit journal, list your feelings about Acceptance.

> **Example:** *Acceptance is constant flow. This is solid. It can be good; it can be hard; it can be bad. But by watching others, I see Acceptance. I know what I can do and can't do. I know the laws and what it takes to be educated. I understand how to talk and know what truth or a lie is. Acceptance is good, whole, right, full. It is knowing what is expected of me. It is "When in Rome, do as the Romans do."*

Next, in your journal, list your guaranteed feelings, feelings that you have a right to. Place the work "guarantee" in the spirit section of Acceptance. Only through Acceptance is anything guaranteed.

Example: Everlasting life—knowing life is always and you are life— fullness, richness, wellness, happiness, and joy are all guaranteed spiritual feelings. Our life is constant flow, and spirit is a constant energy that each one of us has and is able to access always.

Place the word "belief"in the feelings section. List your beliefs about Acceptance in your journal.

Example: I believe in color, energy, and flow. I know that my belief will overcome fear. Fear is an emotion to guide me and say, "Look—what's wrong here?" Through many years of following my vision, I am able to teach and be the Wolf, a path follower, one who shows the path to others.

Place the word "clarification" in the totality section. In clarification, as listed under totality in the mini-wheel of acceptance, we slow life down and look at our strengths and weaknesses. You are in control of your Clarity. When you keep a journal, make plans, set goals, draw symbols, or make mental notes, you clarify. When you stop to clarify, slowing things down to a simple pace, this helps life to be good. List your feelings about clarification in your journal.

Example: When you have totality within Acceptance, you have stamina, the ability to carry on and achieve, to overcome name-calling, being poor, the loss of your job, whatever—and go on. You have the ability to find a place in life to stand, get a job, start over, work hard, and make it happen. Stamina is quiet, being at peace with yourself. The person with self-esteem will listen to the good people speak of him, and will pray and know that Great Spirit hears all prayers. To have self-esteem you build a mental picture and make a list of what you want to have be active in your life. With self-esteem, you can also look to heroes—teachers, parents, and others—whom you see as a good example, and follow their path.

Place Acknowledgment in the concept section of the Acceptance mini-wheel, and list your acknowledgments in your journal.

Example: In planning for a new job, you make lists of where you'd like to work. You list new experiences you need to have for the new job. You look at your ability to go with the flow. This is where you make a list of what you can do or what you want to do. Make a list of things you can't do and need to learn. The ability to go with the flow means you ask questions and look for answers, use the library and read, learn that the world is yours to live. You have good actions, kindness, and fairness. This is where you watch, study, and understand that all things take time. You seek out good advice and keep faith, be kind to yourself and believe. Be fair with yourself and others. Remember things don't change overnight. It takes time. If you do your prayers, have a vision of what you want, and study the success of others, you will get where you want to go. Acknowledgment is to accept that you have hard times, but the concept of Acceptance will carry you on. For example, when the water people came to Turtle Island, there were wars and many were killed, but the race of people who lived there originally are still there and going on to this day.

Go through the mini-wheel that you have built and list your spirit of Acceptance.

Example: *As I sit in prayer and do my prayer ties, I listen for a familiar voice of guidance from Great Spirit. This voice is calm and peaceful, and as I feel it, I am confident. The Confidence brings about Strength. From my communications with Great Spirit, I now am in the spirit of Acceptance.*

List the things you accept. List your feelings of Acceptance.

Example: *Life is hard but I can do anything I set my mind to.*

List your totality of Acceptance.

Example: *Others have dreams and vision, and they make their dreams happen. I can do that too. I will study, work, and I will reach my goals.*

List your concept of Acceptance:

Example: *I see others make lists, seek out teachers, read, and learn. I see others get over fears, and I can do this. I will apply myself and let go of my anger. I can do what I set out to do.*

Knowledge is the secret to success in Acceptance. If you don't know, you can't study, can't do as you are asked. When you get a new job, it is good to be trained by someone at that same job. Knowledge is schooling, skill training, watching others who do and are what you want to be—artist, shaman, wife, husband, mother, father. All of life is a circle of what was and is. "Life goes on" is a good example of the flow of energy known as constant. Great Spirit is constant.

When you work with Acceptance as an emotion, it is an operative force of agreement: As I see I will do. What I don't know I will learn. There are guarantees that if I know it can be done I can do it. If I don't see it done, I can look and ask if it is so. Maybe I'll be the first and others can follow. There is clarification, acknowledgment, belief, support, and meaning. I will look at examples of my elders and wise ones, and I too can have my goals and dreams. Through illumination and study, I will bring forth action, thought, intention. I will put forth the action of movement and understanding.

Use the mini-wheels for the primary emotions and look at the spirit, feeling, totality, and concept of each emotion. Study your emotions, apply Strength, and have Success.

Ceremony of the Red Rose

Tools: *Ground on which to plant a rose bush; rose bush; rose food; peat moss; cornmeal; tobacco; shovel; your smudge bowl, sweet grass and sage, matches; journal and pen.*

The ceremony of the red rose is an honoring of the self. The red rose stands for your Strength. The ceremony is done to celebrate it. The best time for planting the rose is in the spring—the day after a full moon.

1. The opening of the self. Sit with your journal at the beginning of the day, preferably at sunrise, but definitely before 10:00 a.m. The first part of the ceremony is the opening of the self. Allow yourself to look at your weaknesses and list them. See the things you feel most empty, most sad, most angry, and most disconnected about. Find these weaknesses deep inside yourself, bring them out, and list them. They represent the thorns on the rose. They are clues that you are acting out the emotions of fear, sadness, anger, or disgust. It is the rose's way of protecting itself. It is your way of destroying your human connection to spirit by protecting yourself, by allowing yourself to be a thorn. You are pushing yourself away instead of pulling yourself towards.

2. Honor the ground. Choose a piece of ground in which to plant the rose bush—a park, your own yard or someone else's—where it can remain an honor, an achievement. Honor the ground by placing tobacco and cornmeal, and smudging the ground in the area where the hole will be dug to plant the rose bush.

3. The purchasing and the bringing of the plant. It is important to know a little about roses, so go to a nursery to purchase the rose bush and ask questions. Read the instructions and pay attention to what the rose expert tells you to do. Part of gathering Strength is understanding and having knowledge.

4. The opening of the hole. The rose represents the male, and the earth represents the female. You need to re-unite the rose with the earth. From there you will grow your strength.

Start in the East with prayer, and dig a hole in the ground. When you have achieved a hole of the right depth for planting the rose bush (by reading the instructions), place cornmeal in the hole and plant food for the rose. Then place the rose bush in the hole and put in your prayers for Strength by taking a pinch of tobacco and holding it to your heart, making your prayer, and placing the tobacco in the ground. Fill in the area around the rose, packing it loosely with peat moss and dirt. Cover the hole but do not press down on it. Pressing is anger. Just cover the hole lightly and loosely. After you have covered the hole, give it water and watch your Strength grow.

5. First bloom. When your rose bush puts out its first bloom, look into the rose. Spend time around your rose bush; go to your rose bush to pray; go to your rose bush to dance.

If you cannot get to a place where you can plant a rose bush, do this ceremony in your mind. Go into your mind, close your eyes, breathe deeply, and see the rose bush in front of you. Go there in your spirit and be there with the rose. One of the most beautiful things in shamanism is that you can have both the earth and the spirit world. You can go both places and become enriched.

Your Spirit Shirt

Your spirit shirt is a white shirt that carries the seven symbols of the emotions. Each symbol represents not only your emotions, but also your medicines and lessons—the seven medicines of Strength, Success, Vision, Beauty, Healing, Power, and Great, and the seven lessons of Clarity, Poise, Discipline, Account, Fact, Sense, and Complete. In this book you will be given a vision for each level of the Dance. You will be given the Vision of the Elk, the Vision of the Turtle, the Vision of the Hawk, the Vision of the Dragonfly, the Vision of the Frog, the Vision of the Owl, and the Vision of the Snake.

Examples of Spirit Shirt Symbols

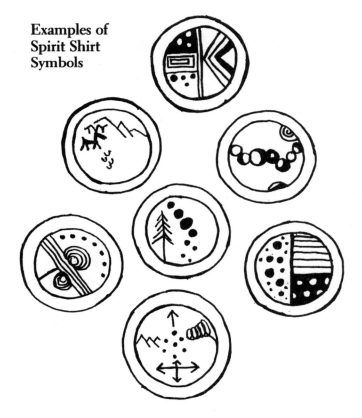

Within each symbol you must bring forth the knowing. Your spirit shirt will help you get to know your spirit better, to understand your primary emotions, the spirit medicines that apply, and the lessons of the emotions—to be open, to *"hold,"* and to *"be."*

In the area of *holding*—to hold is to pray with, to wear, and to know that you understand the depth of this south part of yourself, that you understand your emotions. To *be* is to wear your spirit shirt with honor and pride. You may want to tie colored ribbons on it—or make it an official ribbon shirt by sewing lengths of ribbon to the shirt. There is no right or wrong way. You can apply ribbons the way you want in accordance with your family, your clan, your nation, your belief, your lodge. You can simply be an individual and apply decoration for yourself, which I recommend as the best.

To be open is to wear your shirt and have others say to you, "What is that?" And you say, "Nothing. It's a private thing." And you are open to their words, but you are closed to running off at the mouth. You are select and you are private. When you apply your symbol, make the circles individualistic. Keep the outer rim green, but let the inner circle reflect the color you are working with as you go through each symbol. Use paint, beads, sequins, and glitter—make your shirt very special. For it is *your* spirit shirt. It shows what is in your spirit, what comes out through your emotions—what you dance, dance being live. Wear your symbols with great pride and know that they connect to the lessons and the medicines for each color. Understand that each day you sit with them, each day you listen to them—they will carry their truth to your heart.

Aho.

Spirit Shirt Vision of the Elk

Tools: *A white shirt that is 100% cotton, with no buttons up the front, preferably a T-shirt or sweat shirt, or a shirt that has been made for this purpose. It should be a shirt on which you can sew ribbons and beads, on which you can paint, but the shirt itself should start out plain white. You'll need acrylic paints or fabric paints in the colors of red, orange, yellow, green, blue, purple, and burgundy; smudge bowl, sweet grass or sage, matches; journal end pen.*

Go to a quiet place where you won't be disturbed. Smudge. Breathe in and out four times, close your eyes, and relax. In your mind's eye, in spirit, you will begin to see a path. This path will take you to a lush garden. There you will see a rose bush. This rose bush is beautiful, rich, and full. It is heavy with red blooms and you will see one that is very large. Go to that bloom, place your hand underneath its head and look into it. When you do, you will see your symbol for the Dance of the Red Rose. Don't force it, just look. You may see through thought. You may think, you may see, you may know. Bring these thoughts and sights back, and write or draw them in your journal.

> *Example: I looked into the rose and I saw a line with two dots over it. The line was blue and the dots were red. I brought that back and recorded it in my journal.*

> *Another example: I looked into the rose and I saw a beautiful sunset behind black mountains. I saw four teardrops, one red, one green, one yellow, and one black. I brought that back and journaled it.*

When you are receiving the vision of your spirit shirt, do not think—just be. Do not force it, do not worry—it will be there. It will be a knowing. What you know should go on your spirit shirt for the Dance of the Red Rose.

Your spirit shirt will have seven circles that you may paint anywhere on it. The outer circle of each of the seven circles will be green. For Strength you will paint an inner circle of red inside the green circle. Then, in the center of that you will draw your symbol.

Strength Medicine

It emerges in the sunrise; it *is* the red. It is the life force energy and the blood of the two-legged. When Strength is in movement and its medicine is in its wholeness, it has its confidence and that is its song. Its movement is strong and Confident. It allows the Nurture to be fulfilled. It allows one to give to oneself and to others. It brings about an absolute solidness. It has within it the patience to endure and brings about endurance. It opens the door to all. All movements of life are within Strength—having, giving, taking. Strength medicine is all of these things. Within its personality and in its own character are compassion, mercy, divinity, and respect.

The Process of the Lesson of Clarity

Clarity is a lesson. It comes to you in connection with the hummingbird. Its medicine is Strength. The four steps to this lesson are very simple. Clarity is simple.

One of my elders once said to me that if the watermelon doesn't get water it won't grow. The first step is:

1. Understanding. No water, no watermelon. If we don't have understanding in our life, in our emotions, we are in denial. We are disconnected from the flow we are in. Often in life we think things will be one way and then they're not—they are the way it really is. It's like the watermelon—no water, no melon.

2. Explicitness. The water is 90 percent of the melon. Often the melon is known for its sweetness or its size, when it is the water that makes the melon. It is important that in our lives and the goals of our lives we know the real reason. In the lesson of Clarity, when we accept things for the way they really are, not the way we think, then we have Success.

3. Clarity. The rain is where the water for the melon comes from. We can self-water, carry it in buckets, but however we do it, the melon has to have water. When we and Great Spirit supply water to the melon, the result is a good, big, sweet watermelon. In our lives, if we are clear about where we stand and what our power is, we will reach our goals. A lot of the time, the need for water in our life is overlooked, and we blame ourselves and look to others for our Success. When we are solid on the Facts, we know that water is the key. In our life, to be clear is the key. The whole picture has to be seen and understood.

4. Brilliance. The watermelon got lots of water and the right amount of sun. It has grown to a brilliance. Richness and joy will be the outcome. As brilliance is tested by time, so is the amount of water and sun in the brilliance of the watermelon. When you understand the flow of anything, the outcome will be bright. Your strength is based on understanding the lesson of Clarity.

These are the teachings of the lesson of Clarity.

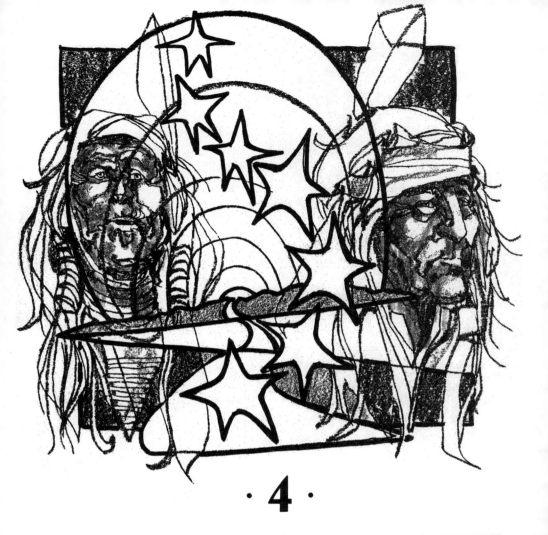

· 4 ·

THE DANCE OF THE EARTH

I breathe in and out. I am stepping from the red stone, the Dance of the Rose, the Red Star of the South, to the orange star next to it clockwise. The drumming is soft, beyond beat, off beat. The students' eyes are full of eagerness. I drift away. I smell the scents of the desert. I smell fresh, opened earth, farm land. I feel sand in my teeth. It hits my skin and I smell the sea breeze. I hear the rushing river, the trickling brook. I am sitting very still, and my spirit is rising higher and higher. I look back at the earth. I see it—a blue, green, and white ball spinning beneath me. I stand very solid in spirit, on spirit ground, looking at the same substances that earth is. It's all red dirt, orange dirt, and yellow dirt around me. The grass is brown. The river moves by fast.

I take a deep breath and let it out. The soft drumming goes on. Before me a path leads me on. I find myself walking within a narrow area. A canyon closes in around me. I see a fire; night has fallen. A flute is playing. I hear the wind swirling around the canyon. The fire throws the shadows of dancers on the wall. As I come forward, I see a tripod with a shield hanging on it. In the center of the shield is a large turtle shell. Around it, on the edges, eagle feathers lie neatly side by side in a circle. The shield is made of eagle feathers and a turtle. In the center of the turtle I see prayer ties hanging—red bundles of prayers.

By the fire I see One who sits cross-legged, hunkered over. I walk close and I can see a person; I see him very clearly—playing his flute. The wind spins and whispers through the canyon, the thunder echoes. As I come closer, I see the One has a turtle shell for a back, the legs of a man, turtle claws for hands. I walk around front and see the human/turtle face—eyes of a turtle, face of a human, nose of a turtle, small chin of a turtle, an extended, wrinkled neck, arms of a man with the shell of a turtle for a chest. It must be a spiritual person playing the flute, swaying back and forth. Before him I see seven bundles. He looks up and says, "Ahh! It's you, Wolf. Oh, yeah, I've been waiting. Sit. Here, let me get you some soup." He takes a rattle and shakes it over the big bowl of soup that hangs on the fire, dips a cup into the soup, and hands it to me. "This is earth soup. It's made from all the brothers and sisters, all the things that walk and crawl. This is in honor of all places. When you eat this, it will open up your heart."

He sticks out his long willowlike fingers with turtle claws on them and says, "I'm Turtle Heart. Eat from my brothers and sisters, and listen to the story of the earth."

I sit down beside Turtle Heart and look at his face, withered and wrinkled, old and distant, eyes a piercing yellow—round and vibrant, yet with a soft look. He waits and watches as I eat. At first my mind drifts, hoping the soup will disappear, because what is *in* it? I look, and there is everything in it. When I look in the bowl I can see the river; I can see trees and deserts, sky and ocean. I blink my eyes and look again, and I see a brownish-looking stew with lumps of meat and what look like vegetables of some sort. Oh, well, it can't be any different than anything else in spirit. I take the soup and start to eat quickly, hoping it won't taste too bad. Ugh! Horrible-tasting stuff! Ugh! Gollee!

"Heh, heh," Turtle Heart laughs. "Disgust! Isn't it disgusting? Isn't it wonderful? Don't you find offense in it?"

Ugh! He is ugly. His piercing little face is looking right at me.

"It's worse than that! It's sickening, it's horrible!"

"Hmmm," he says. "Hmm. Earth can be that way, you know. It's a sickening, disgusting, annoying place. Don't you find it that way?" He glares at me with his piercing little face.

"Well, I find certain things that way." Ugh, I can taste the dirt in my teeth. "What is *in* this stuff?" I say.

"I told you. Earth. Everything. My brothers and sisters," he says. "If you could eat it all, it would be a great success. Now *that's* an interesting word. You would have attainment. You would have great victory and wealth. You could count coup on all your fears. Yeah. You could touch 'em, get command of 'em. You could count coup on Disgust."

Hmm. I'm beginning to get dizzy. My stomach is starting to spin.

"Oh, that's just disapproval. That's just you not wanting to do it." S-l-o-o-w-l-y, he begins to move. Very, very slowly he reaches for a cup of soup, and starts eating it.

Oh, my head is spinning. Things are getting very s-l-o-w. Very s-t-i-l-l. Noises feel like pins sticking in me. "Oh, I really dislike this." An extreme hostility begins to roll over me. All around me things are becoming very, very orange, very, very hot. He begins to play the flute again, and it pierces me. Each note seems to be burning into me. Unh!

He stops and says, "Drink the rest and achieve Success." His words fade in and out.

I take a deep breath and I feel myself in the fire. All around me are flames and heat. I eat the soup. I take it down, the foul taste, the stench, the dead feeling in my body. I cannot stand the sounds of the flute any longer. "STOP!" I cry out.

He looks at me. "You have achieved Success. You have done what you were told. It is my medicine to open you up to the Earth."

"Well, if that is truly the Earth, it is hard for me to be open," I say. "It isn't easy for me to look at the Earth and think of anything nice most of the time. My job deals in misery and sorrow. I listen to pain and agony. It is mine to bring the message. I am the path. I am the teacher of Rainbow Medicine. I carry the vision of the sun, the moon, and the seven stars." I feel the annoying sickness passing.

"I have a great deal of disapproval, very strong disapproval, for what I see on Earth," I go on. Mankind has been about murder, war, and indignity. Brotherhood and sisterhood should be like a circle—it should be in peace, a sacred hoop. I have been told this by my Grandmother and Grandfather Wolf."

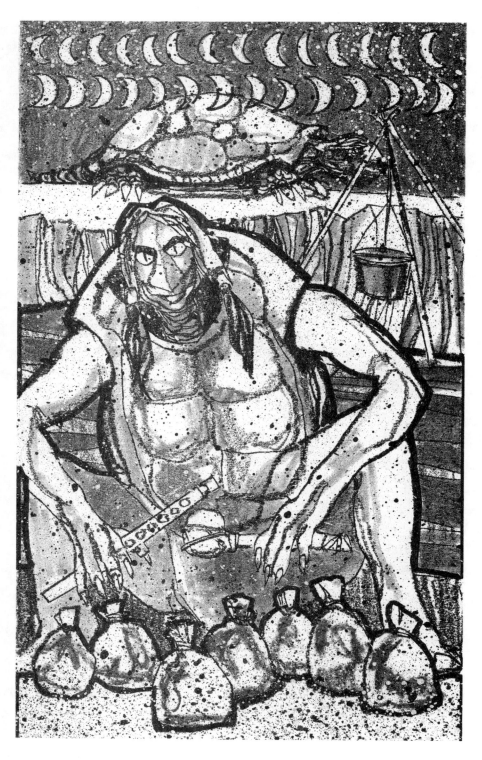

"Oh, yes. I know Grandfather Wolf. He lives by the river, where my kind grow. Many turtle people. They walk along quietly on the Earth, telling the story of Steadfast, my great-great-grandfather. You see, Steadfast once went to war with Stubborn. Stubborn was an old hound dog who tried to bite his head off. But my great-great-great-grandfather just pulled his head back in, slowly and methodically. His victory was in his stability, his ability to get calm, his ability to regain his Poise. He was quiet in his steadfastness. And the old, Stubborn hound dog slapped him around like a rock, batted him around, took him back to camp where there were brother and sister hound dogs, other Stubborns. They slapped him around all day, banging his shell against rock after rock, tumbling him down hills, but he slid out underneath the tree by the river.

"The Stubborn old hound dogs got tired and went on about their way. Oh, my great-great-great-grandfather laid there—quiet, quiet, quiet. Remembering the lessons that he had learned from Otter. His brother and sister Otters brought him the teachings of grace. How swiftly they moved through the water! How beautifully their bodies slipped through it! How calm they were as they moved through the creek. Their stability, their steadiness—Steadfast remembered those lessons. He became strong.

"It is within the Earth's endurance that the sun comes up and the moon comes out. But there is Success. Within the two-legged there is the emotion Disgust. I have let you taste that today. It is within my Turtle Heart to offer Steadfast, the victory and wealth of Success.

"The earth is a story of Success and on my back lie thirteen spaces, one for each moon. It is the blue moon, the second moon of December, that is the thirteenth space on my back. The story speaks of many secrets, for it is said that we have twelve months, that we have twelve signs. But there are thirteen moons. The second moon that is full in December—where does it come from?

"Look," says Turtle Heart, turning to the sky. I look out and see four red moons, four orange moons, four yellow moons, four green moons, four blue moons, four purple moons, and four burgundy moons. Casting their light in all the colors, they have risen. There are twenty-eight moons."

"Wow—how pretty! But why so many moons?" I ask.

"Well, there is one for the spirit in each color, one for the emotions in each color, one for each body in each color, and one for each mind in each color, to guide and teach the path of life, the Sacred Circle," Turtle Heart says. "Twenty-eight moons, Wolf. One day, when you get to the Great Falls, where you meet up with your Grandfather Wolf again—good friend of mine—he and Grandmother Wolf will share with you a deepening, an enriching from the Great Falls. Your Success is based on your attainment, your victory, your wealth, and your coup. When you count coup, you face your fear, look it in the face and learn, touch it and walk on," Turtle Heart says.

"I don't want to touch my fears—I'm too angry at them," I say. "They weaken me, and I never win. I'm too scared of them to touch 'em."

"You must remember what you tasted," Turtle Heart says. "To be offended, to dislike, to be repelled—two-leggeds spend much of the time in this kind of hostility, disapproval, displeasure, sickness, and annoyance. It is time—it has long been time—that you walk past this.

"You draw from the moons—they are the mother teachers," Turtle Heart goes on. "They give you their teachings of Success, Strength, Beauty and Power, Vision and Healing—that's the way to count coup. Your Elk medicine—Strength, the color red—is waiting to help you draw on the energy of the color and stand solid."

I look at the beauty of the colored moons. What a sight! What a feeling!

I look around me. Turtle People, many of them are sitting around us, rattling, most with soft drums and flutes. They all are playing different songs. The wind swirls. The fire turns everything around me orange. I watch the sparks of the fire join the sky. I see trillions of orange stars, scattering.

"This is the Dance of the Earth, Wolf."

I watch them shooting and sparking from the fire to the sky. Turtle Heart shakes his rattle.

I hear the soft sounds of the stars, calling me back.

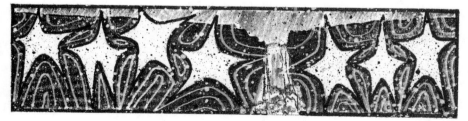

The Emotional Teachings of Disgust

Build a mini-wheel for disgust. In the center, place a stone for disgust. On the right, in the spirit position, place a stone for repel. At the bottom, for feelings, place a stone for annoy. On the left, for totality, place a stone for sickness. At the top, for concept, place a stone for displeasure.

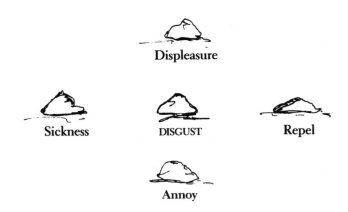

Displeasure

Sickness   DISGUST   **Repel**

Annoy

When working with the teachings of disgust, you'll need to open your spirit journal and list all the things that repel your spirit.

Example: Darkness, abandonment, absence, empty.

These things repel the spirit and bring about the emotion of disgust. Make a list of the things that you feel have repelled you in a spiritual way—of the places where there is darkness and emptiness, loneliness and sadness, abandonment and neglect in your life.

Example: A young man has had a very rough life at home, exposed to lies, anger, alcohol, violence, drugs. He was abandoned for long periods of time and left alone for whole weekends. From the age of six he was left to take care of himself. Now at age 17, he dresses in black, painted his room black, took his bed out of his room, and replaced it with a coffin to sleep in. He has no expression in his eyes, no goals for his life. He hardly goes to school and has changed his name to "Dark Heart."

In feelings, make a list of things that annoy you, things that cause aggression, anxiety, nervousness, apprehension.

Example: A little girl is sitting on the school bus. The boy behind her puts gum in her hair. Her aggression builds because of her anger, and she finally turns and slaps the child behind her, starting a slapping match. This causes anxiety in the bus driver. First a nervousness comes over her because she fears that things are getting out of control. Her anxiety builds and finally she yells at the kids and keeps yelling to get them to quiet down. Apprehension grows in the other kids because of her anxiety, and they join in the fight. Soon everyone is yelling and fighting, causing the driver to have to stop the bus and settle the matter.

In totality make a list of things that make you sick within the totality of disgust, such as uneasiness, hatred, rage, bitterness, denial.

Example: A teacher knows that a student is writing hate letters to people. She discussed it with the student, but it does not stop the mail. The teacher has a strong uneasiness because she has said all she can to show the student the point she is making. She can see hatred in the eyes of the student and a building rage, but the student is in deep denial. She tells the teacher bitterly, "I'll write what I want when I want the way I want." The student quits, calling the teacher "alien" and other names. There is no way for the teacher to clear the matter until the student faces her own rage, accepts her feelings, stops her hatred of herself, and lets go of her bitterness and her need to hurt others, as she was hurt herself.

Under concept, make a list of things that bring displeasure to you, such as laziness, ignorance, arrogance, stubbornness, closed minds.

Example: An artist sits and watches his colleagues becoming well known. He wants to have money and sell his work, to be famous and have people worship him. He is very arrogant, and he doesn't listen to people who tell him he has to work harder and try different approaches in his work. His arrogance keeps him from accepting that people need to like him and his work in order for him to achieve what he wants. His ignorance won't let him hear. He feels everything he does is better than other people. He is stubborn and closed-minded. He doesn't work on new ideas but steals ideas from others. These attitudes keep the artist away from the Success he seeks, and cause loss of his relationships as well.

Remember when working with the mini-wheels of the emotions that you can use them for any topic to which disgust is connected, or for any topic to which any of the primary emotions are connected. Set up your topic and then follow it through your mini-wheel. This allows you to open up and express yourself in the four quadrants of an emotion. Be sure you state the topic at the top of the page in your journal.

Example: In disgust, I feel connected to my failures in relationships.

Then you can review your relationships and see where you repel or feel repelled, where you have annoyed or feel annoyed, where you have felt sick or displeased. Then you will see the total four directions of disgust as they apply to your relationships.

Aho.

Ceremony of the Earth

Tools: *Sage; sweet grass; tobacco; 4 yards (3.6m) of red 100% cotton cloth; sea salt or plain salt; cactus seeds or other various types of flower seeds; cornmeal; a small bottle of water; red yarn or cord; smudging tools; paper and pen.*

The ceremony of the earth brings forth bundles of prayers for the earth. You will be bringing one for the ocean, one for the river, one for the city, one for the desert, one for the mountains, one for the trees, and one for the sky.

First, find a quiet place where you won't be disturbed. Cut the cloth into 12-inch (30cm) squares. The first bundle you make will be for the sky. In the sky bundle you will place prayers. Leave the first cloth square open and think your thoughts into the sky for cleanliness, for healing. Place the bottle of water on the cloth. Then fold the right corner over to the center, the left corner over on top of the right corner, bring the bottom corner up and then roll the bundle into the top. Tie the bundle in the center with four knots. Mark it with a strip of paper that says sky, and set it aside.

The second square will be for the desert. In this bundle you will place sage, plus cactus seeds or sagebrush seeds or any desert plant seeds, plus tobacco and cornmeal. Place your prayers for the desert in the bundle. See the desert staying in balance with its beauty, with its dryness. Close the bundle as before, folding the right corner over the center, then the left corner over the center, then bring the bottom up over both and roll it into the top. Tie it in the center with four knots, mark it "Desert," and set it aside.

The next bundle will be for the trees. Lay cornmeal on the cloth with sage, sweet grass, tobacco. Say prayers for the trees, for the standing people that they may continue to grow and always be amongst us. If you wish, place seeds for trees or a small tree in your bundle to be planted. Close it by bringing the right corner over the center, then the left corner over the center, then bring the bottom up over both and roll it into the top. Tie it in the center with four knots, mark it "Trees," and set it aside.

The next cloth you will fill with tobacco, sweet grass, sage, and corn-meal. Put prayers into it for the city, that the city can be clean, that the people can be happy, that things will come about in a good way, that the cities will get better. Bring the right over the center, then the left, the bottom up over both, and roll into the top. Tie it with four knots and mark it "City."

The next bundle will be for the mountains. Place prayers for the mountains in your bundle, for them to continue to be a safe haven for the four-leggeds and the winged ones, for the trees and the wind spirits. In this cloth you will place flower seeds, little seeds for trees, or any other seeds of plants that can grow wild on the mountainsides. Add sage, sweet grass, tobacco, and cornmeal. Fold the right over the center, the left corner over the center, bring the bottom up over both and roll into the top. Tie in the center with four knots and mark it "Mountains."

The next bundle is for the ocean. Fill this bundle with sweet grass, sage, and sea salt and pray for the ocean to become clean and healed, and that people will learn to respect it. Close the right over the center, the left over the center, bring the bottom up and roll into the top. Tie with four knots and mark it "Ocean."

The last bundle is for the rivers and the lakes. Place sweet grass, tobacco, and cornmeal on the cloth. Place prayers for the purity of our rivers and lakes, for their healing. Fold the right over the center, the left over the right, bring the bottom up over both and roll up into the top. Tie in the center with four knots and mark it "Lakes and Rivers."

Sit with your bundles and make a list of things you can do. (1) Clean up around yourself and everything you own, and get it in a good way, so it is clean and bright and good. (2) Plant living things, flowers, seeds, plants, and trees. (3) Plant just a tree or a bush. (4) Go to the ocean, the river, the lake, and walk. Carry a trash bag and clean up as you go, taking care of the banks of the rivers and the lakes and the ocean. (5) Walk along the roadway, out along desert areas—anywhere that is in wide-open country, and clean the sides of the roadway, picking up trash and litter. (6) In the city, paint, clean away trash, offer to haul off trash for others, do windows, and clean up graffiti. Wash down sidewalks. Put out trash cans. Pick up trash and put it in trash cans when you see it. Bring a pride to your city by smiling and waving and saying hello to others.

Sit with your bundle and think about these things. Try to do something once a month for your world, for the Earth. You are her arms and legs. Take time from your busy life and apply your goodness. Bring your Beauty Way to the Earth and bring her Success, so that she can live on for generations and generations.

Take your bundles to the places marked upon them. If it's marked to go to the city, take it to a place in the city where it can be burned, and burn the bundle, letting the prayers rise up to Great Spirit. If it is for the sky, open the bundle, open the bottle of water, and throw the water into the air, representing the cleanliness of the air, washing the air clean. Dispose of the bottle properly. Place the red cloth in your medicine wheel to remember your prayers for the sky. The rest you can bury. Dig a hole, open the cloths, and let the seeds go to the Earth. Place your ocean and water bundles on the water and let them float away, allowing the water to become one with the cloth and the cloth to become one with the water; in this way you are bringing the Earth and water together.

This is the Ceremony of the Earth.

Aho.

Spirit Shirt Vision of the Turtle

Find a quiet place where you can sit. Close your eyes, relax, and breathe in and out four times. Before you, you will see a path. Follow that path in your mind until you come to a nice, grassy place, a place where you can sit on the ground. Have a tree beside you. Breathe in and out. You will feel yourself become very solid and heavy. Let your spirit rise. Feel your spirit leaving your body, going up. Feel yourself rising above the trees, up into the sky, above the sky. Look back. When you look back at the planet, you'll see your symbol for the Dance of the Earth. Remember it and bring it back. Record it in your journal; then place it on your spirit shirt by drawing a circle in green, a second circle inside of that in orange, and placing the symbol inside of that. This is the spirit shirt vision of the turtle.

Success Medicine

Success is the medicine—the orange stone that you place in your medicine wheel. Success is attainment, it is victory, it is coup, it is wealth. Make a list of what you need to obtain in life. What are your attainments? Make a list of what your victories are, what you have taken victory over in your life. Where have you won? Make a list of what your wealth is—what makes you wealthy.

Example: The spirit of your dog, the beauty of the grounds you live on, the sky that you draw breath from.

If you want, you can include the money you make, but always remember that it is not the objects that you own or the money you possess, but the blessings you have. Here, in wealth, count your blessings.

Next, what have you counted coup on? This means, what have you faced.

Example: It took a long time to become a writer. There was much turmoil and many twists and changes in my life. But my profession announced itself and I became a creator, an author.

Count your coups, what have you faced? The fear of losing a limb? The fear of being locked up? The fear of divorce? The fear of death? Count your coups, that you have faced them. Each time you count a coup, you hold a feather, or you can make a star, to place on your coup stick.

Coup Stick

Tools: *A stick 5 to 8 feet (1.5 to 2.4m) long; a leather string (or another type of cord); decorations, such as animal representations, beads, paint, bells, feathers, stars, red cloth.*

Cut the stick from a green tree so that it is still alive and pliable. Bend the top approximately one to two feet (30 to 60cm) in the shape of a candy cane—long and in an arc at one end. Tie one piece of string or leather to the arced tip and the other end to the stick itself. This will keep the stick in the candy-cane shape. Then decorate the stick by placing a represenation of your clan, your family, or your favorite animal on it. The decoration can be skin or cloth that is the color of a certain animal that is your clan. You can bead, color, or paint symbols on the stick that represent the coups that you have counted. Tie bells on it; it is appropriate to tie four bells for each coup that you count. Draw circles all over to represent the joys that you feel. Prepare feathers by wrapping the end of the feather (where the quill is) in red cloth; tie it four times with pieces of string, and then hang the feathers on the coup stick. The coup stick will look like this:

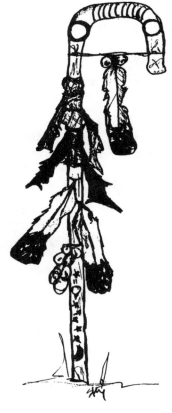

Coup Stick

Every time you count a new coup, add a feather or four bells to your stick. Each time you touch your enemy, each time you look your greatest fear in the face, each time you achieve and bring about Success is a coup. For each accomplishment, each achievement, each victory, each prosperity, each time you thrive—bring it forth and place a symbol on your coup stick.

When your stick is finished, hang it on the wall of your home. If you prefer, and if you have land or a yard at your home, you can dig a hole and stand the stick in it upright. Bury the bottom six inches (15cm) of the stick.

The Process of the Lesson of Poise

Poise is Otter Medicine. It is a lesson that will help you stand always in Balance. Balance is a Spirit Medicine and Poise is a lesson of the emotions, a lesson from Success, a lesson that you must learn in order to obtain Success. In having Poise, you look Disgust in the face by knowing what is disgusting to you. Follow these four movements to obtain your Poise:

1. **First is grace.** Grace is the ability to let go and move with a smoothness. Write down your smoothness: things that you are stable with, things that bring you a good feeling.

2. **Second is calm.** Moving through grace, it brings a calm into your life. Calm is brought about by letting go, by forgiveness, by dismissal—by sitting in the wind and being quiet.

3. **Third is stability.** Stability is a knowing, your ability to bring forth your solidness. Stability is a connection of calm and quiet. Prayer brings about stability. It is the result of knowing that you have been heard by and are valuable to Great Spirit.

4. **Fourth is perseverance**—being able to keep on, to achieve, to accomplish, to have victory, and to count coup.

When you have brought these movements into your life and you can list them and journal them every day, then you have learned the lesson of Poise. This gives you strong Turtle Medicine, allowing you to understand your Disgust, disapproval, displeasure, sickness, annoyance, dislike; what gives you offense; what repels you; what your hostility is about.

It is important to open your heart of Success in the completion of the Lesson of Poise. A Success is to be looked at here as solid, knowing what you believe and need. Have a plan, set goals, for this brings Poise to a full expression. Poise is also the act of being organized and steady.

Aho.

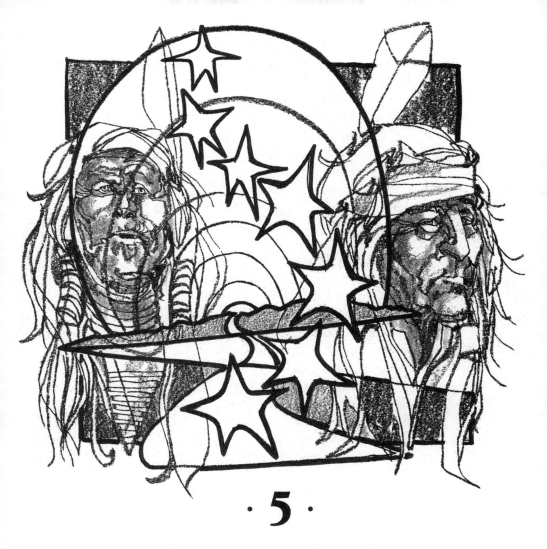

· 5 ·

THE DANCE OF
THE YELLOW BIRD

I breathe in and out. I relax. I continue breathing. I am sitting quietly, looking out over the hill at small candles twinkling. Ten vision squares are laid out. Spirit lights are dancing around, glimmering. Green ones there. Red ones over there. A soft mist comes over the visions. The beauty of the northern lights, soft swirling colors. I see the Milky Way. Its spiral comes closer, the stars swirling, making a path. A small yellow bird flits past me, following the Milky Way. I begin walking on the stars, through the mist.

I find myself traveling along a dirt road. A quietness blows through the wind. The tall yellow grass sways back and forth. I come to two old cottonwood trees; they must be hundreds of years old. Their yellow shimmering leaves sparkle in the sunlight. I see a fire, a campfire. I see a camp. There in the yellow grass I see extended wings, a man dancing, a bird spinning around and around—one and the same. I move closer and stand behind a big rock. I look up, over the rock, and watch.

The man is bare to the waist; his arms are the wings of a hawk. His tail is yellow hawk feathers. His legs are those of a man, but painted yellow with white stripes. Around his ankles are bird fluff and feathers. Moccasins cover his feet, beaded with bright yellow beads, close to gold. He has tiny golden bells attached to his moccasins. As he dances, he flexes his wings. His face is part human and part hawk. He has one yellow eye, and one beautiful green human eye. His skin is reddish brown. He is strongly built and square jawed. There are black, yellow, and white stripes over his rib cage.

His camp is very comfortable. A buffalo robe is his bed. His food is all neatly stacked around the fire, pieces of meat that look to be rabbits and squirrels, skinned and properly stretched on sticks. His wood is stacked and bundled. Prayers and feathers hang in the tree. The wind blows softly and the smoke spirals around.

He stops, and brings his wings down to his side. "I have been expecting you, Wolf." His voice is clear as the sky. "I understand that you are on your way to see your Grandfather Wolf, who will be meeting you at the Great Falls. Sit with me, and we will talk."

I step close to him. A frequency shift has taken place around me. Color sparks off his feathers. He has changed. He stands barefoot now in blue jeans, a man with a long braid down his back, with hawk feathers tied in his hair. He wears a necklace with hawk talons, and in the center a hawk's foot. It hangs over his heart, to the middle of his stomach. He wears other necklaces of gold and beads of yellow, made from corn. His hands are well formed and beautiful. One eye is yellow and one eye green. His face is beveled, strong, and muscled in his jaws. He sits on a stump and asks me to sit beside him. I sit on the ground and lean against the rock.

"This is a wonderful home. Gee, I don't even know your name."

He looks at me and I can hear the thunder rolling across the plains behind him. The sky turns misty yellow. "My name is Hawk. Yellow Bird."

"What a beautiful name, Hawk Yellow Bird."

Above me a red-tailed hawk circles. It whistles. The center feather from its tail floats down over our heads, and lands at Hawk's feet. Four small

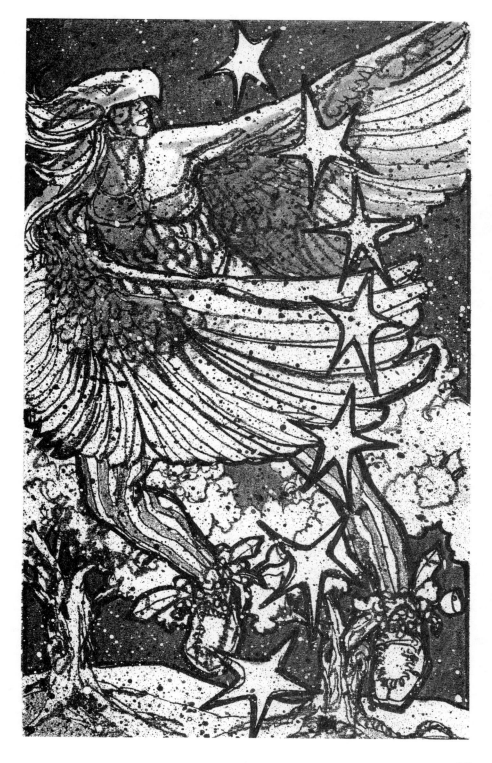

yellow birds land on his shoulder. They are yellow finches. I become very tired. I feel myself fall backwards into the mist.

"You must stretch out, Wolf. Lie on the buffalo robe."

I lie back on the robe and look up into the sun. It is white. I can hear the hawk whistling above me. Yellow Bird begins to rattle. He rattles quickly. It sounds like the tail of a rattlesnake.

"It is mine to give you Happy, Wolf. I hold within me, in my heart, the symbol of Happy."

I open my eyes and he is standing above me. Out of the solar plexus area of his body flies a butterfly—a beautiful, yellow butterfly. It spirals around and around and around. "Butterflies are the discipline. They are the symbol of the sacred hoop of life."

The one butterfly becomes many, and they all fly about and become stars. As they do, each one of them turns into a song note, a musical note, and I can hear it. Each one of them pops open with joy and sounds of happiness, notes of music.

There is much delight in my heart. I have never felt so cheerful. I have never felt so satisfied. The noonday sun warms my body. The quiet of positive thoughts are solid in my mind. He rattles slowly. The rattle gets slower and slower, and the sounds of the stars that the butterflies bring forth become singing wind. I watch the wind blow through his hair. I watch him change into a hawk before my eyes, and he flies around, circling higher and higher.

"It has been your discipline, Wolf, to carry forth your vision."

I look to the right, and he is sitting there. Evening has come. The butterflies sing on into the evening, soft rattling. He has rebuilt the fire and it is flickering.

"Your vision has brought you much discipline. Its training has become your practice. Its development has brought your course. It is through your vision, the voice of your dream, that your spirit emerges. I will tell you now of the Dance of the Yellow Bird. It is insight. It is perception. It is a time when you prepare to go within a sacred square. Each student is called to see Great Spirit. It is mine, the Yellow Bird, to open your heart to the song of the butterflies. You hear the song of the stars, Wolf. Don't you?"

"I hear the wind calling me, always. I hear its twinkling sounds, its rushing sounds, Hawk. I hear it call me out into the evening, and into the morning. There is always a joyful sound."

"From the Seven Stars you have come here, to the Green Gate, facing the Emotions."

I smell the summer evening turning to night. I watch the sky become a darker shade of blue. I listen to his words on into the darkness. He speaks of my perceptions. He speaks of my understanding, of following my spirit, listening to the sun and the moon, listening to the father and the mother, the bearers of great happiness.

"Do you remember the nightmare, Wolf? Do you remember the sparks of gold that fought with gentle splashes of silver? Do you remember the gift of the woodpecker, when he pecked the holes within the wood? When he gave us the gift of the flute? And how the sounds of the song did not come until the wind graced the holes he had pecked within the wood? Can you remember those things? Can you remember the songs of sorrow, of sadness, that blow through the evergreens and live evermore? Do you know what that sadness is about? It is within your vision to bring forth your knowledge."

I am alone. In the quietness of the morning the sun has risen again. There is no camp. Just me. I am sitting inside a square of golden cord with four white flags that blow in the breeze. The hawk circles overhead. I simply sit with the sun and the moon, and the seven stars. And I remember.

"I do remember, Hawk, the nightmare. I remember the loss of happiness. I remember abandonment and grief."

At that moment, four yellow horses with golden auras come up over the hill and start grazing. They come from the North. The yellow bird flies past me and lands in a tree, singing a sweet melody.

"It's not far to the delight of your heart, where you will be pleased and satisfied always. You will sit with your Grandmother and your Grandfather and you will hear the stories of Great. Keep with you the memory of family, always. The tradition of Grandmother and Grandfather, mother, father. Remember the Discipline, the things that you have been trained in, the development of our course, Wolf."

I listened to the yellow bird sing and the hawk whistle. The trees are alive with yellow birds. It is the song of my vision, sweet birds singing in the morning, the soft rattle in the night, the image of the sun, the crescent moon, and the seven stars. I hold it always as the sacred seven teachings.

I hear the soft sounds of the stars calling me back.

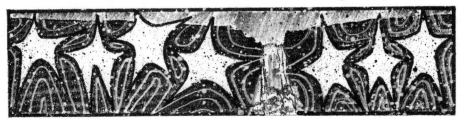

The Emotional Teachings of Happy

Make a mini-wheel of Happy by placing the emotion Happy in the center. The spirit stone represents satisfied. The feeling stone represents positive. The totality stone represents fruitful. The concept stone represents delighted.

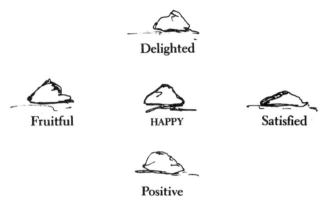

Delighted

Fruitful   HAPPY   **Satisfied**

Positive

List what is satisfying for your spirit.

> *Example: Prayer. I feel a fresh start when I connect with Great Spirit. I like to use prayer ties when I pray; it allows me to clear fear and anger from my mind. In the act of prayer I feel clean and organized. I have a bright, fresh outlook afterwards. To me "bright" is hope and faith. "Fresh" is excited and happy. Both feelings give me the courage to go on. Going on with life is satisfying to my spirit.*

List your positive feelings of Happy.

> *Example: I go for a walk in the woods and encounter the spirit of the trees. The tree spirits are alert and healthy, and this brings great happiness to me. While I walk, I hear the cheerful voices of the bird people. I am filled with gladness because of their gleeful sounds. The sky is clear and allows me to see the spirit of the mountain in all its grandeur. The mountain brings joy to my walk. As I complete my walk, I come to the point: as my spirit comes face to face with the spirits I encounter on the walk, they and I all have a positive feeling of Happy.*

List what is fruitful for you in your totality of Happy.

Example: I studied with a teacher for several years to learn true spiritu-ality. He had me do many tasks, such as naming my achievements, explaining my hopes, and knowing my Wisdom. I spent years getting the answers to his questions, and came to the conclusion that my wealth of friendship, my prosperity of family, and my hard work in life are my blessed achievements. The years with my teacher and finding the answers are a totality of Happy. Spirituality is fruitful. And it must always contain forward motion. Listening to the voice of my teacher and gaining understanding is fruitful for a totality of Happy.

List your delights for the concept of Happy.

Example: When I do spirit work with people, a lot of the time I sit in prayer and clear my mind of all judgments. I keep an open mind on whatever matter the person is dealing with. I might spend hours or weeks alone in this thought process. When I return to normal physical life, I am very happy to come face to face with others, my family, my dog, my friends. All of my family, my dog, and each friend I have is a true delight. In relationship with each one in my personal circle, I gain tranquility and enlightenment.

These are the teachings of the emotion of Happy.

Aho.

Ceremony of the Yellow Bird— Building a Vision Square

Tools: *100% cotton yellow cloth, cut into one-inch (2.5cm) squares, 400 of them; four poles that are 4 feet (1.2m) tall, made of wood— you'll paint one pole red, one green, one blue, and one white, red for the spirit, green for the emotions, blue for the body, and white for the mind; paint in all seven colors, red, orange, yellow, green, blue, purple, burgundy or seven colors of string or yarn that you can use to paint or wrap your poles; four pieces of 2 × 24" (5 × 60cm) long white cloth; 36 feet (10m) of yellow cord or yellow yarn or string; a knife or scissors; journal and pen.*

With the knife or scissors, cut four pieces of the white cloth—two of them 6 feet (1.8m) long and two 12 feet (3.6m) long.

Sit quietly, taking the time to make 400 prayer ties with tobacco in the center of the yellow cloth squares. As you do, ask Great Spirit for your vision, to give you an answer, to show you the place where you are to go to do your vision, and to instruct you as to the person who will sit with you quietly and watch over you. It is recommended that you seek out a lodge leader who can take you into a sweat lodge. If it is possible for you to do this, it is important to do it traditionally and in a good way.

When you have completed your 400 prayer ties, start preparing yourself for four days prior to your vision. I recommend that you fast with fruit juices only for those four days. You will need to pray for 24 hours, on the fourth day of fasting, from four in the morning to four the next morning. While you are praying, ask to speak with Yellow Bird and to be shown your vision guides, the four guardian animals who will stand with you at the four poles. As you are in prayer, you will know the four animals. Remember them and put them in your journal.

In the middle of the fourth day of fasting, go to the place where you know your vision square will be. This must be outside, in a place where you will be undisturbed. I recommend a place on private property where you will be safe, with no interruptions. Make sure that it's okay to hold a spiritual ceremony there. The person selected to accompany you will sit and watch, be in prayer for you, and keep anyone from bothering you.

Prepare your square by digging holes and placing the four poles in the ground, one in each direction—East, South, West, North. Tie your cord to all four poles, making a square. Tie the four flags onto the cord. The cord is there to provide safety in spirit for you. It lets the spirits know that this is a ceremonial spot. The flags are there to call the spirits in.

To prepare to go into your vision, enter the vision square at 4 a.m. You will stay there for 24 hours. You are not to leave the square for any reason. You will be carrying with you your 400 prayer ties.

At sunrise, you will string 100 prayer ties onto the east section of the cord. At noon, you'll string the south section of the cord with prayer ties. In the evening, you'll string the west section of the cord with prayer ties, and at midnight you'll string the north section. Each time you do this, offer up prayers to see your vision. At midnight, you'll lie down quietly, knowing that your vision will come to you, knowing that you have your four animals guarding you in the four directions. Rest until four in the morning. Then cut open the cord on the East and walk out through the East, rolling the

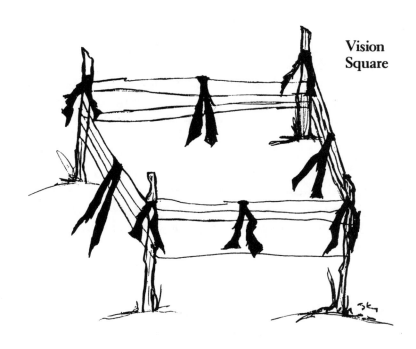

Vision Square

cord up all the way around. Then walk around again and remove the poles. Then build a fire with the poles and prepare to meet the sunrise. By this time, you will know your vision. You will see it in a symbol and know it in your mind. It may be that you will have to return to your vision square often, because your vision has not been clear to you. Or you may not have understood the depth of it. Each time you wish to go, tie your vision square, sit within it, and listen.

Aho.

Spirit Shirt Vision of the Hawk

Find a quiet place where you can sit down. Have your spirit journal with you. Breathe in and out four times and relax. Lie very quietly on the ground, eyes closed and breathing softly. Open your eyes and you'll see a hawk flying in a circle above your head. Remember, this is in your spirit sight. Look inside the circle where the hawk is flying, and you'll see the vision of the Yellow Bird. Bring back that symbol and record it in your journal. Paint a circle of yellow on your shirt, inside a circle of green. Place the symbol—the vision that you saw from the Yellow Bird—in the center. This is your spirit shirt vision of the hawk.

Vision Medicine

Vision is a simple circling of knowing. It is through the lesson of Discipline, through going forward and looking, that you have Vision. Vision is an opportunity that comes from the noonday sun—from the solid brightness in your life. It means opening up your heart and allowing yourself to see things within the simple, having the Discipline to understand that life is more than what someone tells you; it is what you see and know with your own spirit's mind. You bring the Vision forth in your life by simply knowing what you see. Vision medicine is very strong within Discipline, for you must own what you know. You must see it and you must listen and bring it forth. It is the opportunity to know what Vision medicine is.

The Process of the Lesson of Discipline

To obtain a vision, you need preparation and discernment. Discipline is the lesson needed to obtain your Medicine of Vision. There are four steps in the process of the Lesson of Discipline.

1. Clearing, dismissal, forgiveness. Allow yourself to understand, to be whole. You must understand Acceptance: that things are the way they are and you may not be able to change them. You can ask if they can change. Ask yourself, the people involved, a teacher, doctor, or others involved.

Understanding Acceptance allows for clearing. Often, just understanding the rules or boundaries helps you reach Acceptance. Allow yourself to understand Disgust: this will help with dismissal.

When you are disgusted, it means you don't want it—the way things are. You don't like the way things are. When you have disgust and accept it, you "let go." Dismissal happens. Much of the time we two-leggeds need to accept that life isn't going to go the way we want. Allowing yourself happiness and joy, you open yourself to feeling large and full. Clearing is then at hand. When you have these feelings, the flow of energy is at hand. Allow yourself to feel anger and you will see you are closed—shut down. Allow fear and this is also a closing of the self, not knowing which or what to do. Your training in understanding and allowing the emotion to teach you is a training brought forth by your choice. The Discipline of the emotions has given you lessons so that you can understand how to cope.

2. Training comes in the second step—practice and journaling. Whatever you do in life with Discipline, you must practice! Prayer is a Discipline—the Discipline of talking to Great Spirit and listening for answers. It may sound like you're talking to yourself, but Great Spirit's lessons will be shown to you, and you will know and hear them in your own thoughts. Action—which is doing—is very important in Discipline training. Within Rainbow/Star Medicine, understanding the Rainbow Medicine Wheel is a must—it is the Discipline of walking the wheel, knowing the words, and seeing the words alive and active in your life. It is the Discipline of prayer, journaling, sitting in the wheel and knowing where you are, the Discipline of learning lessons and knowing what lesson you are in.

3. The third step of Discipline is development. To practice Discipline as an outcome shows you understand and have brought action to be your Discipline. Prayer as an action is an example. Also the understanding of your medicines and using them in daily life is an example. Living your talk, using your knowledge of Power medicine is an example of Discipline. Applying the emotions of Happy and Joy to your life by sharing and caring for others, by being able to forgive and dismiss are examples of Discipline training. Use your mini-wheels. Learning the lessons within the circle of teachings in this program is Discipline training:

Strength: your ability to keep going
Success: opening yourself to mistakes and achievements
Vision: seeing clearly and making a list of what and where you want to go. See what you want as clearly in your mind as a picture on your TV screen.
Beauty: the understanding of others' examples, the lives of the animal kingdom, color and feeling, safety, and happiness within the self, among elders, children, and those who support you.
Healing: the understanding of the sacred circle, that nothing is sick and everything in your life is a lesson. Understand the lesson and you have the cure.
Power: You are Strength, knowing. You have your Vision and understand the voice of your Vision. You apply your Acceptance of your emotions and use the Disciplines of Rainbow Medicine.
Great: Great Spirit will always be your faith. Great is Great Spirit, that you are alive and life is great.

Even though it is hard at times—hard is a discipline—it is important to be cheerful, even if you can't or won't make what you want happen. To count coup, and touch your fear or anger, will bring you a satisfied, pleased feeling of delight. If you want Success in Discipline training, work harder. Study the words in the Medicine Wheel and bring them to action in your life.

4. Which brings about the fourth step, which is course. The course of your life is obtained by looking at your training. If your training is in anger and hate, then your practice will be anger and hate, and the development will be your demise. If it is in goodness, and justice, and right—then you will obtain the practice of goodness and justice, and your development will be a course of action that is cheerful, satisfied, pleased, and delighted. The emotion of Happy will reign. You will have the ability to have your vision at that time, when your perception, discernment, insight, and mental image are clear.

Often Discipline can come in the form of the physical: the training of how to eat, how to exercise, how to obtain what you wish to practice in life. It is up to you to bring about your course of life—through education, through growing strong in your elders and in their wisdom. It is important to listen to the tradition of your family. It is important to dig deep within the roots of your family, to go to what is you, to open the door and find the depth of your emotions, the things that make you angry and sad, the things that bring about fear.

The process of the lesson of Discipline may be developed in many different ways. It is up to you now to make the process of the Lesson of Discipline a teaching.

Aho.

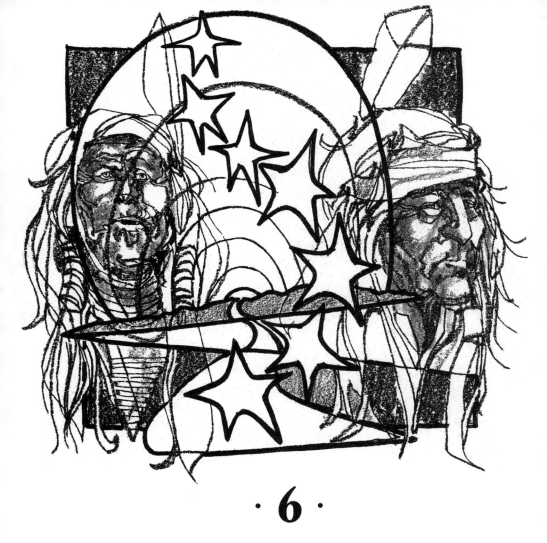

· 6 ·

THE DANCE OF
THE EVERGREEN

I breathe in and out, and continue breathing. Quietly I rest and I breathe.
Before me I see a sparkling trail. It moves along the ground in an "S" shape,
weaving its way back and forth. The sun hits it and it sparkles, millions and
millions of tiny points of light. I walk on the sparkling light on the trail of
the thin line. It leads me along within the forest. I see curly, ruffled ferns; I
see Boston ferns; I see others—all types of ferns. And trees, enormous

pines, huge cedars, fallen logs that must have been there for a long, long time. I smell the fresh earth in the dampness, the different kinds of moss, and the tiny trail keeps taking me along its thin little line of shimmering, glistening color. Over the logs, along it goes. I come to a rock where the thin line disappears. This rock is a nice place to sit in the afternoon sun and rest. I sit on the rock and study the little trail that I have followed. It is that of a snail. Hmmph, it is that of a slug! For there in front of me *is* the slug. He looks at me. He is green, with black spots.

"They refer to me as the Banana Slug, here in the forest. Why have you come here, are you sad?"

"No, I'm not sad."

"This is a place where people come to deal with sad, and more often than not they come here with broken hearts. They are grievous; they are bitter. A lot of the time they don't have a spirit when they come here—they are so empty and heartsick. They come here and they walk—they follow the trails. I see them a lot, the two-legged; they walk through the woods and I know they are Sad because I see their tears. Most of the time, though, they see me as ugly. Do you think I'm ugly?"

Hmm. I look at the little slug. He is a nice size—he's funny—but he radiates Beauty all around him. There is a presence of greenness about him that is assuring to me.

He twitches his little antennas and he promises me, "I'm not ugly, but here in this place, anyone can find ugly. Look there, there are the snarled ones. Look there, there are the twisted ones. Look there, there are the weathered ones. I have my purpose."

And he begins to scoot along, to creep along, to move along, disappearing beneath the leaves, leaving his little shimmering trail of thin.

It is odd for him to ask me if I am sad. It is more than sad that I have come to the forest with. In the coldness of life I have learned many lessons. I begin to walk through the forest listening to the sounds of the winged ones, the cracking of the sticks, and the wind softly blowing through the pines. Since the Slug brings it to my mind, Sadness is there—the emptiness, the coldness have swept through me like an empty hallway.

Before me I see an enormous tree. It is as wide as an automobile. As I start walking closer to it, I can see it has a door in the trunk. The door bursts open and the light pierces me, a green, vibrant light. The light is beautiful; it is the fullness of Beauty in every way. I stand there, feeling the warmth of the light, receiving all the blessings it might hold for me. And before my eyes is a unique creature. She is a combination of all the woodland spirits— a brownie, gnome, and troll. She is the most beautiful thing I have ever seen, fair and small. Her eyes are reddish brown and they twinkle. Her hair is the same color like the bark on a ponderosa pine. She is dressed in tight green skin. She has no shoes, but her feet are bark, that curls at the toes. Her hands seem human, but when I look closely, I see they are pine branches with little pine needles for fingers. She wears a shirt made from all types of leaves.

"Good afternoon, my name is Jack, and I am the Spirit of the Tree."

She can fly. She lifts up and circles around me and, as she does, she sheds tiny green stars. Her laughter rings out.

She says, "I know. You have come here and been accused of being Sad. Going for a walk in the Beauty, just simply admiring the charm of the forest. Don't let those things bother you. Don't let the Sadness that the Slug speaks of slow you down. Don't let things that are grievous, bitter, or painful ever slow you down. You have come here to the forest to listen to stories of charm and fairness. You have come here to receive the blessings of the Beauty of the forest."

She sprinkles more green stars on me and, as she does, I feel weightless. "Come with me, and I'll show you."

Lifting with her, I fly! I take flight as a dragonfly. The wonder of it! It isn't every day a wolf gets to fly! I am no longer a wolf, I am a spirit within the green.

We move up and out through the top of her home, and from limb to limb all through the forest. I see the splendor and the fairness of the animal kingdom—how they take care of their kind. I see the tender, loving tongues caressing the cubs. The blessing of the forest is its quietness. As we fly, it is so quiet you can hear our wings moving.

"It is here among the Standing People that you are in the family of Beauty. It is here within Beauty that there is breath—it is the most wonderful thing there is, to breathe, to have life in its fullness," she says. "As Jack, I am the Spirit of the Tree. I am the Spirit of the Evergreen, living forever here in Beauty. For our roots entangle and entwine and we live always as one, for we came from one seed and we are all one, together. We all share the same, be we the apple tree of love; or the poplar tree of support; the pine tree of life; the oak tree of strength and solidity; the maple tree, the most beautiful, the one that shows the cycle of life; be we the strong cedar, the ever-present tree of blessing, of ceremony, of cleansing, and purity; or the evergreen that lives on forever. We are all Standing People. We have all come together as our roots work their way deep within the Earth Mother and unite.

"Welcome to the forest, Wolf Moondance. We are so glad that you have

107

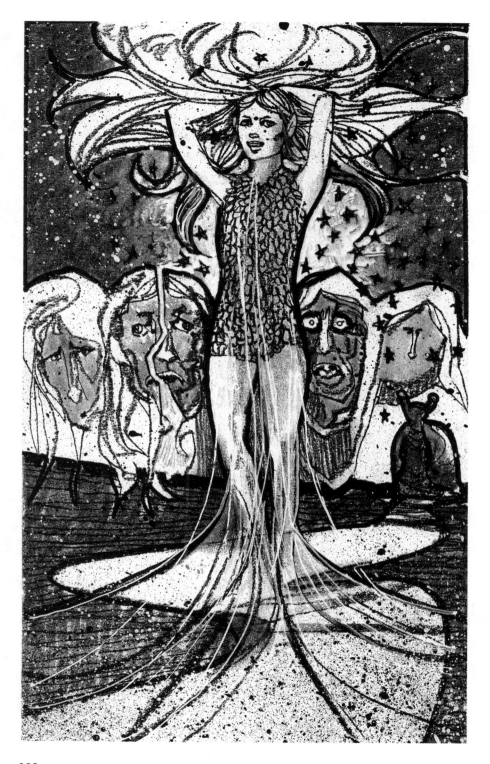

come here to feel the quietness. Today is the day that you will learn to sit with it, like a rock. Today is the day that you learn to be solid within your walk. Come with me and I will show you."

She returns me to the ground and I can walk again. My life is normal. The forest is like a familiar rock.

"Here, sit here. Sit here now, and look within the Circle of Sad, for it is in those feelings that your bad choices are often made. It is from Beauty that you will be healed. But before that time comes, before Healing Medicine is in its fullness, you must understand charm, fairness, balance, and blessing. To do that you must look within the ugly of yourself."

I sit surrounded by green; it is all around me. Jack disappears in the twinkle of a star. I hear her voice very quietly say, "Sit still. Sit with it, like a rock. Become solid and quiet. Understand the Discipline lessons and bring about the solidness of Account. For the Slug has opened the door and has given you the opportunity to understand Sad."

It begins to rain, and a mist falls. As the mist grows heavier and the plants drink, I become empty and quiet. I can feel the brokenness, the Sadness, the sorrow filling my heart. I feel myself as a rock. I become very solid and drenched in wetness. It is the bitterness that wakes me. Why is it that I am to sit in all this Beauty and feel Sadness? How can Beauty exist within Sadness? Or Sadness within Beauty? As the evening wears on, I become the rock. I grow heavier and quieter and deeper. I become the ground. I become the roots of the Standing People. And I, my spirit of wolf, follow the entwining, winding, turning path of the roots deep down within the Earth. I fall into a place, deep within, down, way down. A place where I sit and it is quiet. There is a circle of spirits around me.

One looks at me with eyes that point down in a long willowy face. "I am Sad." Another looks at me with one eye going one way and one eye going the other, and a face that is split. "I am Broken." One looks at me with a blankness and paleness deeper than death itself. "I am Grievous." One looks at me with a pointed nose and sharp, beady eyes. "I am bitter." One is wrinkled, saggy, and sort of slouched. "I am Pitiful." "The rest of us are dispirited," and I look but there is nothing there. "Heart sick," and it is so faint that I can hardly see the face. "And sorry," the saddest and most pitiful of all.

They are faces, and nothing more. They are a circle, a council of faces. They sit in their grievous, bitter, broken way and moan a chant. They sing, "Ho he, ha ha, ho he, ha ha." A mockery they have brought. From the center, a spiraling, colorful band of light emerges, swirling its way down to the ground in the circle. There a little fire bursts out, and tiny green spirits that look like flames and stars jump from it. There are pale ones, dark ones, medium greens, hints of yellow and blue, and they begin to dance. They call out, "We are the spirits of Charm. We are the spirits of Fairness. We are the spirits of Balance. We are the spirits of Blessings." As they dance, they drop little seeds. "We are the beginning of life. With all our Beauty we dance and sing. We push back the sad, the broken, the grievous, the bitter, and the pitiful. We dance on sorrow, we dance on the heartsick. We dance on the dispirited and bring them to life."

I watch the dance move on its way. I watch the flames of the fire spread and cleanse the faces.

I take a deep breath and I am sitting at a campfire. In front of me is a wonderful person. She has long brown hair; her eyes are soft brown; she is fair. She is dressed in all the radiance of the forest with a green cape, green skirt. She has a medicine bag in which she carries antlers, rocks with holes, pieces of wood that she has carved into small animals. Her bag is beaded with berries and seeds in intricate patterns of greens. Her smile is devious.

"Do you have a name?" I ask.

"Oh, yes, I have a name," and she raises an eyebrow. "I am Grandmother Evergreen—Jack's mother. I am forever life. Within me is fairness. I wish to give you that gift."

She reaches out her hand, and I take what she gives me. It is a small green feather.

"Hold this forever in your fairness. Understand that all the ugly that you have seen in your face will break you and it will bend you, and it will make you bitter." She extends her hand and gives me a rose quartz star. "Hold this star. Place it in your heart and keep it, for it is your balance." As I take the star, I see it is tinged in orange—radiant orange light. "Hold this star within your heart for balance, always," Grandmother Evergreen says.

She then pulls from her medicine pouch a long strand of green and silver. It is green beads and silver stars. She swings it in circles and, as she does, it makes a sound—a song cascades around me. "Charm. You must have your charm, dear." She holds it lightly and hands the chain to me. "When you are no longer in your fairness and in your beauty, when you feel that you are pitiful or that you are broken, you are sad and you are bitter, sing with this chain and listen for your charm. You must look at the charms of the stars and hold them in your mind's eye. For silver is that of spirit and it twinkles in the night, in the forest, and we all hold that in our minds. It is a large part of being ever green." Her eyes twinkle.

At the moment that she says "ever green" I see behind her the spirit of the coyote passing from tree to tree, beckoning me, trying to get me to feel disconnected. I hold on very tight to the charm that she has given me and do not turn to see what trick King Coyote offers me. I take a deep breath and understand that Sad is a choice among the emotions—that I have the opportunity to feel Sad at any time. And I also can choose the feeling of Beauty—that Beauty is a medicine that comes with all of its charm and opens the door to fairness.

"You are learning. You are learning. The lessons are not easy, for you must go deep within the dark underworld and confront the faces of ugly always. Within yourself there are always things that separate you from your beauty," Grandmother Evergreen says, "but remember this," and she pulls out a tiny tree. "Plant this tree and be ever green. Put Jack in the earth and let her grow."

I look into the face of the tree and there is a small dragonfly. She emerges and flies around me. As she flies, she sprinkles tiny green stars and bright bouncing green lights.

"You have received the blessings now, of Beauty. The blessing of Evergreen has come to you. Walk in the forest always, and be amongst us."

The wind swirls around me and she is gone. But I can hear her song in the trees, in the song of the Standing People sharing their voices. It is great to be with Grandmother Evergreen and feel her Beauty. Her lovely reddish brown hair, long and flowing with flickers of darkness and light—I hold in my mind. The stillness of the rock lesson will always be mine, for it is a good thing to walk in the forest and take a thought, and sit with it like a rock. I know that this is my blessing.

I hear the soft sounds of the stars calling me back.

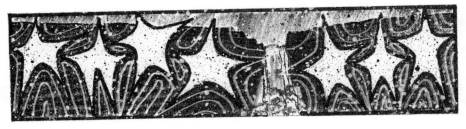

The Emotional Teachings of Sad

Make a mini-wheel for Sad by placing Sad in the center. In the spirit put Grievous; in the feelings put Bitter; in totality put Pitiful; and in concept put Broken.

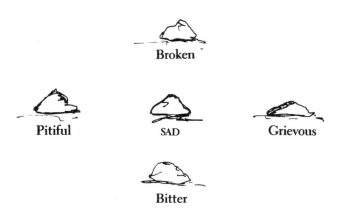

Broken

Pitiful

SAD

Grievous

Bitter

Take your spirit journal and list the things that are grievous to your spirit in the emotion of Sad, such as abandonment, death, disconnection, lying, denial.

Example: People are put here on the Earth Mother to live, and life is a circle; we learn this from those around us. A child is slowed down in life when it is abandoned. The child is going to feel fear, and is going to have a loss before it can get a good start in life. When the child goes to school, it will not care, and its self-esteem is affected. It will feel discouraged and will not learn as well as the child from a home of solid parents. Homework will not be done and the child will lie and say that the homework didn't get done because he or she was sick. Or the child will go into total denial and say things like someone stole the homework, or that a chore had to be done for parents. The child can come to a point where not even death affects the level of feeling going on. The death of a good friend may happen, and the child doesn't care at all, or claims not to. All of this comes from abandonment. The emotion is Sad, lonely, empty.

Within the feelings of Sad, list your bitter feelings, such as gossiping, backbiting, belittling, anguish, and despair.

Example: A divorce has taken place, and the man involved is very sad. He goes around to all the couple's friends and talks with great anguish and despair because he can never have the relationship back the way he wants it. He tells people how much better he is than his ex-wife, how the only way she knew was to quit and give up 20 years of relationship. He talks about her behind her back wherever he goes, telling lies, belittling her. He gossips about every problem she has or has had to anyone who will listen. *It is important to remember that all this is taking place because he is sad. The sadness expresses itself in actions of bitterness.*

Within the totality of Sad, list the pitiful thing, such as depression, mental anguish, denial of your mental state, and emptiness—leading to abandonment, harmful actions, and mental illness.

> **Example:** *A couple loved each other for over 20 years. She used drugs and drank alcohol excessively. He was a heavy pot smoker. She called off the relationship after going for help. He became very hostile and came to her house, hit her, kicked her, and performed other harmful actions. He packed all his camping gear and headed off to hide. The sad feeling got worse. He stayed away, but the emptiness and denial of his mental state got worse. He went to a bar, bought dope, and started up again. Finally, after weeks of mental anguish, loss of sleep, loss of appetite, loss of job, leaving his children, and many other pitiful acts and events, he turned himself over for help with the mental illness of depression.*

List the concept—Broken—of Sad, with such things as broken heart, attention-seeking, aggression, anxiety, spitefulness, and despicable thoughts, spirit and mind.

> **Example:** *A friend of mine went to see a counselor because she had such aggressive feelings and behavior. She had cut her hair with a knife. She was anxious, always thinking everyone was talking about her. She called our friends and said spiteful things on their answering machines. She was a despicable mother. She wouldn't even take her child to the doctor for medical help. She claimed most of her problems were caused by a broken heart, which I define as a misunderstanding or making the choice of feeling sorry for herself. Her Sadness was the driving force behind her broken thoughts. She couldn't keep up with work or family requirements. Her spirit was broken, she said, and that's what pushed her to do bad things. She spoke of a broken mind, when in fact she was an attention-seeking person, a condition brought about by having been put up for adoption as a child.*

Work with your mini-wheel of Sad and understand that Sad is broken and grievous, bitter, pitiful, spiteful, dispirited, sorry, heartsick. Work with the areas in your life where you practice the emotion of Sad. What brings you to that spot? List the things that make you bitter. List the things that bring sorry into your life. What is sorry for you?

My advice within each mini-wheel is to look in the dictionary, and copy out the synonyms and antonyms of each word. Get familiar with your language and understand your actions. Am I Sad and broken? Am I grievous? What brings me to these states? Own your mini-medicine wheels. That means to take them on and understand that as a human, as a two-legged, you have emotions and you have choices. Will it be sadness or acceptance? Happy or sad? It's up to you.

Ceremony of the Evergreen

Tools: *Spirit journal; pieces of paper; a place to build a fire—a fireplace or fire pit; wood to build the fire; matches to start the fire; a small evergreen tree to plant; shovel; a place to plant the tree.*

The Ceremony of the Evergreen brings about Beauty Medicine. Beauty is charm, fairness, balance, and blessings. It can shimmer and shine; it can sparkle.

1. In the Ceremony of the Evergreen, the first thing to do is look for the ugly in yourself. When looking for the ugly in yourself, apply honesty. And remember it's within yourself, from yourself—what you think of as truly ugly. Ugly is repulsive, ugly is *less than*. Ugly is not good enough. Ugly is blackened, hardened, turned-away-from, closed, disconnected, and denied. Look for the ugly within yourself, such as habits, addictions, actions, and motivations.

2. Look at what makes you Sad. Sad is broken, separated from, abandoned, neglected. Sad is bitter, spiteful, sharp, hateful, sorry. List the things that make you sad. Remember that Sadness is beyond tears; it's deeper.

3. Build a fire—preferably a campfire—but a fire in a fireplace is possible. You will be placing evergreen boughs over the flames. If you are doing the ceremony in a fireplace, only burn a small piece of evergreen. If you have a campfire, have a large pile of boughs.

4. After you build the campfire, place the things that you have written that

are ugly and the things that are your sadness on the fire with all of the evergreen boughs.

Watch the smoke rise and see the colors in the smoke. Read them. Do you see blue or orange? Yellow or red? Or just white? Read the colors. Look them up in the back of the book.

> **Example:** *If the smoke is yellow and blue, then* Vision *and* Truth *are my answer—or* Vision *and a need for* Healing. *If the colors are orange, red, and white, there is a need for* Strength *and* Success *in my spirituality.*

Let the papers that you have burned become pure ash and let the fire go out. Record every color that you see—physically or spiritually—from the time the ceremony starts. Interpret the colors and read your message from the Ceremony of the Evergreen.

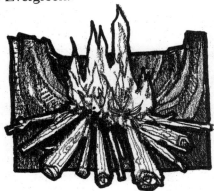

5. The last step in the Ceremony of the Evergreen is to plant an evergreen tree.
   a) Buy the tree and find the ground in which to plant it.
   b) When you have bought the tree and found the ground, the second step is to open the ground. Dig a hole with a shovel, as advised by the nursery where you bought the tree or the instructions that come with the tree. Place sage, sweet grass, cornmeal, and tobacco in the hole along with plant food for the tree.
   c) The third step is to place your tree in the hole.
   d) The fourth step is to close the hole and pat the dirt softly and gently around the tree.
   e) The fifth thing, now that the tree is planted, is to water it generously. Pray for your Beauty that, within the Ceremony of the Evergreen, you will always have it, and for the lives of the Standing People. Pray

that a tree shall grow and give you breath, bringing forth your connection to Beauty.

Gather rocks—one rock for love, the connection to the Earth. The second rock is for the energy that comes from the tree to the two-legged. The third rock is for the power to the air, that the tree gives fresh air for us to breath. The fourth rock keeps you connected, solid, gives you roots on the Earth and the understanding that you now have family; you are connected to the Standing People. Place these four rocks around the base of the tree. Allow the tree to grow and go often to see its progress. Know that you are building Jack the Tree a new home and know that all of the Jack spirits thank you for their homes. Go there and allow your energy to be connected to the Earth; feel your energy run up and down from Earth to sky to Earth.

This is the Ceremony of the Evergreen.

Aho.

Spirit Shirt Vision of the Dragonfly

Find a quiet place where you won't be disturbed and sit with your spirit journal. Take four breaths, relax, and let go. Let your eyes close. Before you, you will see green grass. There will come a dragonfly. That dragonfly will lead you on a path, walking through the grass. The dragonfly will be your path. You will follow it and it will lead you to a tree. As you look at the tree in front of you, you will see a door—a door in the tree. Open the door. When you do, you will see your symbol of the Dance of the Evergreen. Remember your symbol and bring it back; write it in your spirit journal. Draw a green circle within a green circle and place your symbol in the center. Transfer the symbol to your spirit shirt.

Herb Bundles

Herb bundles are blessing bundles. They are made for house blessings, protection of the self, for the aroma of the herbs that are within, and to give you Strength and Beauty. Bundles are meant to overcome and to balance sadness. They are made from herbs and cloth, tied with sacred cord or string in the colors that bring about the teaching within the bundle, or to bring Beauty, charm, and blessings to your life. They are to bring Balance. This is the Beauty Way.

There are many ways to make herb bundles and many different kinds of bundles for different purposes. The bundle I am talking about is one that you can place beside your bed, or up over a doorway, or underneath something. You can also make your bundle smaller so you can wear it around your neck inside a medicine pouch.

I would like you to make four bundles. The first one is a house blessing; the second, a protection for the self; the third, a Beauty Bundle; and the fourth, a bundle to overcome Sadness.

Tools: *Your spirit journal and pen; four pieces of green cloth 4 inches (10cm) square; cord to tie each bundle together—it should be red to represent the good Red Road; cornmeal; juniper; pine; piñon; sage; sweet grass; tobacco; cedar.*

You can find most of the herbs in stores around your area, or you can go for hikes and find them. Piñon can be found in the states of Colorado and New Mexico; juniper grows in many different states in the West. Cedar grows in most people's yards. You can buy cornmeal or grind corn and make your own. Sweet grass is sold in many health food stores, trading posts, herb shops, and rock shops. And you can use all varieties of sage. The one that works best is white sage from California or the normal burning sage called "scrub sage," which grows in the states of Washington, Wyoming, Montana, and the Dakotas. You can also find many herbs and sweet grass at local powwows and other ceremonies held by Native Americans. If you do not have the herbs or cannot find them, you'll have to wait until you get them. No substitutions are possible.

After you have cut your four squares of green cloth, hold the first one in the air and draw down the blessings of Beauty. This bundle is for a house blessing. It is there to bring about Beauty in your home. Think of the things that make your home full of charm, full of fairness, full of Balance—and bring blessings to your home. It would be a good idea to list these things in your journal so you don't forget. Place these thoughts into the cloth and lay the cloth down. Place broken pieces of sweet grass on the green cloth. The sweet grass will reduce your anxiety and bring about a centering in your home. Place some pieces of juniper, shavings from the juniper bark, and pieces of green juniper. This herb removes negative energy. It is the protection that drives off and dispels negativity. Place some sage in your bundle; this is for cleansing and honoring. Fold the right sides of the cloth over the herbs. Fold the left side on top of that. Take the bottom and fold it up over it and roll this up into the top. Take your red string and wrap it around the bundle four times and tie four knots. The fours are to represent the directions of your ceremony. Take a piece of paper and write "House Blessing Bundle" and slip it under the ties. Place the bundle to one side.

Herb Bundles

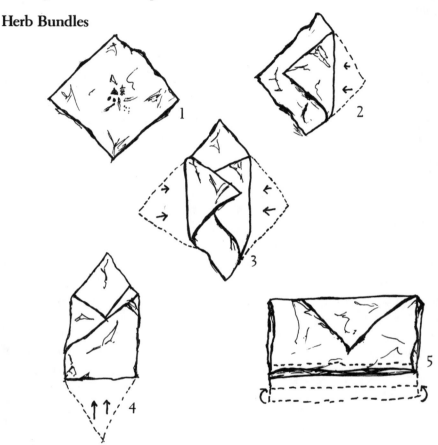

The second green square is to bring forth a bundle of protection for yourself. Sprinkle this bundle with cornmeal to represent and set sacred space, so that the energy fields will be positive. Place some cedar in this bundle—it centers fear and anger. Know that you are protected and centered. Put a little sweet grass there to reduce your anxiety and to bring about balanced energy. Bring the right corner of the cloth over the herbs and the left corner over the top of that; bring the bottom up over both of those and roll it into the top. Wrap the bundle four times and tie four knots to represent the four directions. Take a piece of paper and write "Protection of Self Bundle" and slip it under the ties. Place the bundle to one side.

The third is your Beauty Bundle. Lay your cloth down. In this cloth you can add several other types of herbs and flowers. It is always good to put flowers in your Beauty Bundle—rose petals, carnation petals, daisy petals—all different types of dried flowers, and it's good to add lavender and shavings of sandalwood—both types of aromatic herbs bring about scents of beauty. Place juniper and cornmeal in your bundle. Juniper will remove negative energy and cornmeal will set the sacred space. Place a heavy amount of sage to bring about honor. For Beauty is honor of the self. Bring the right corner up over all the herbs, then the left corner on top of that. Bring the bottom corner and pull it up over that and roll it up into the top. Wrap it four times with the red string and tie it with four knots. Take a piece of paper, write "Beauty Bundle" on it, and slip it under the ties. Place it with the others.

For the fourth bundle, take the last green square. This is a bundle to overcome and balance Sadness in your life. You'll want to sprinkle cornmeal to welcome spirits of the light, to know that you have found guides, helpers, and spirits to help you walk in the light. When you put the cornmeal on top of the cloth, take a deep breath in and think of the colors. See each one of them as a star and know that you have the medicine of Strength. For Strength, put just a little piece of juniper in your bundle. Know that you have Success. For Success put some tobacco in your bundle, and know that you have your Vision, that you can see in the spirit, and that the spirit world is real. Put some sweet grass and sage in there, for your Vision. Take a deep breath and relax. Place some pine in your bundle, for the Standing People, so that you have Beauty. For Healing put some cedar in to center fear and anger. For Power put some piñon in, for piñon protects, cleanses negative energy, and welcomes light spirits. For Great, place juniper in your bundle. It will move negative energy to give protection to your spirit. Fold the right corner of the cloth over the herbs, then the left over that; pull the bottom up over both and roll the bundle up into the top. Wrap it four times with red string, and tie it with four knots for the four directions. Take a piece of paper and write "Bundle to Overcome Sadness" and place it under the ties.

Place your House Blessing Bundle up over your doorway by pinning or taping it, or tie it over the doorway. Place your Protection of Self Bundle underneath your bed. Place your Beauty Bundle where you go every morning to start your day—to brush your teeth, comb your hair. Your last bundle, for Overcoming Sadness and Having Balance—keep on you. Each time you find yourself wanting to be sad or having something to be sad about, balance yourself by holding your bundle and drawing in the beauty from the herbs. And know that you have the blessing of the herbs within your life. The Herb People are the oldest teachers that have ever lived, and they are bringing their sacred ways to your heart through the herb bundles.

Aho.

Beauty Medicine

It is in the early evening, as things start to calm down from the day's sun, that most Beauty happens—in the sunset. Likewise, most Beauty appears with the sunrise, for Beauty is a cycle. It is to Account, to understand the depth of the full cycle of the day, that brings about Beauty. That there is a beginning and an ending, a fullness within all things—this is Beauty. Beauty is not measured by physical means—it is not hair or eyes, it is not measured by what you own. It is energy set in balance that brings about Account, which is the flow. When you bring things to Account, you solidify them, you put them in a place where their Strength is in motion, so that they are a Success. Beauty is the formation of all solidity. It is *all* that brings about Beauty. In all the Beauty that you have seen, you are looking at the face, you are looking at the breath, you are looking at the solidity of Great Spirit.

The Process of the Lesson of Account

The green lesson that is given to us in Rainbow Medicine is Account. Account is your words. It is your word, your reason, your worth, and your self-esteem.

1. The first step in the process of the lesson of Account is to list the words that are yours, the words that you stand on.

Example: Creativity, Impeccability, Truth, and Real. These are the words that I walk with.

List your words—words that are you. Put down the meanings of the words, the ways in which you use them. Examine the words that are you. Make sure that they are the words you want to Account with, that you have to have represent you. If you find words you don't like about yourself, Account those words. Take to heart what you don't want and replace it word for word. When you Account, you should feel good about yourself, but what you list should be true.

2. List your reasons for living.

> **Example:** *I have come to this earth to teach, to be a teacher of life, to give out an example of the good Red Road the best I can, to put to sleep the myth of evil and bad.*

List your reasons. Look for your reasons. If you don't have a reason, then develop one. What are your reasons for being?

3. List your worth. In listing worth, you have several areas to cover.

> **Example:** *My financial statement, my intelligence, what others think of me, where I have been and what I have learned.*

It is important when you are listing your worth that you look all around you for those areas such as what you own, who you run with, who you were raised by, what their qualities are, what your qualities are.

4. Your esteem. Within esteem there are seven things to look at, to ask yourself about.

> **Value:** What matters to you? Family, job, what others say?
> **Cherishing:** Who are your loved ones? Mother, father, granny, friends?
> **Honor:** Your knowledge, what is your knowledge base? Education, teachings from elders, books read, college?
> **Revere:** To what do you show respect? What things have you earned—titles, positions? What things are revered by you? Adored? What things can't you live without—things that you feel are what make you who you are—your job, your studies, your marriage, your children?
> **Praise:** Teachers, other people and things that have taught you, such as Christ, school, parents, loved ones, Great Spirit?
> **Exalt:** The things that exalt you are those that you worship, those that lift you to the highest respect. This should be your God/Great Spirit/Creator.

Take each one of these and list what it means to you. When you have this list, you can see what brings about your self-esteem. It is complicated because our emotions are connected to one another. If we step out of our emotional plane into our spiritual plane and ask the same questions, what we value will be *spirit*, what we cherish will be *spirit*, what we revere, adore, praise, and exalt will be *spirit*. If we brought that back into our emotional plane and danced it through our lives and lived it, then we would bring spirit into our emotions, and we would live that in our relationships. We would show it in our everyday experiences, through the things that we list under our self-esteem.

When you move through the lesson of Account, your word, your reason, your worth, and your self-esteem become the directions of Account, too.

Aho.

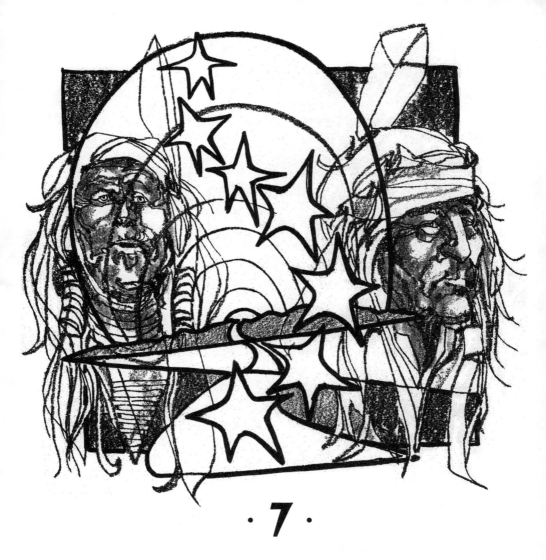

· 7 ·

THE DANCE OF THE MOON

I breathe in and out and relax. I continue breathing easy and slow, and before me I see a silver shimmer. It hits the ground. It provides a path of silver for me to walk on. I follow this silver, walking alongside the river. The silver shimmer is the song of the moon. It hits the water; it hits the ground. I am walking and thinking. I'm letting go. I feel a wave of intensity come over me. It takes my breath away. I feel it tear into the heart. I want to hurt. I feel the rage and the rampage, the yearning, the passion. I look out across the water and I remember—broken promises. I remember when you said you wouldn't promise, ever. I remember when you said you didn't believe in promises. It's a good thing that there are no promises, for you cannot carry them; you cannot fulfill them.

I have taken part in this two-legged walk now for a long time. I am no longer nineteen. I am clear within the dance of life in my emotions, and I have listened to Water Elk. Acceptance is the way. But I have no acceptance for those who have broken their word. It is best not to promise at all if you cannot keep your word. But to manipulate, we sometimes say things so that we can get what we want. It's really stupid. We reach out, grabbing for things that are not ours.

Ahead of me I see a silvery silhouette with long, flowing hair. When I get closer I can see a woman with silver skin. Her clothes are threads of silver, made of tiny silver beads, tiny silver coins woven together into a silver gown. Her eyes are so blue they are silver. Her features are soft and pointed. She is very, very old, yet her face is young. Her eyes dance with spots of stars. In her silver hair are tiny stars, twinkling and dancing. The silver turns to all colors. At the end of each strand of hair is a star.

She looks at me with a softness. "I recognize you, Granddaughter. I recognize you."

In the quiet of the night the silver shimmer arcs above her. "Remember me? I am Grandmother Moon. The fullness of my name is Grandmother Blue Moon. I am the full energy of Grandmother Moon. The stories of Mother God are mine to give.

"I see your pain, granddaughter. Anger is your emotion. You have become passionate. Your passion comes from being annoyed, from your feeling of not being good enough. You are disappointed—the disappointment of being human. It can be explosive, Granddaughter. You must be careful. Your touchiness can lead to belligerence, and you will be full of violence. You must understand that the softness of the water can wash away the passion, the rampage, the wrath. You must join this healing circle tonight. Wolf, when your students come to you in pain and you work with them, their pain is left with you. I see that you hold in the pain and it brings you great sadness. Come with me. I will teach you. I will show you the healing circle."

"I think of the word healing a lot. I think of it for my students and I think of it for myself."

"It's a good thing that you have walked here to me, along the river in the moonlight. It's good that you have come back to talk to me."

"Grandmother, if I were to go to the healing circle, could it do anything about my broken heart?"

124

Grandmother smiled. "It is mine to oversee the affairs of the heart. It is mine to see pain and to bring you to the point where you have choice, where you can either die or mend that broken heart. It is mine to teach you where you made the wrong choices, to tell you that you are very touchy, to explain to you how explosive your thoughts have become, for it is the emotion of anger that a broken heart is." She links her arm in mine. "Come and sit with me by the river where I live. Remember you can always find me there—and at the lake and the ocean also. I shine down on all courses of ebb and flow."

We sit on the rocks alongside the river.

"A broken heart is anger? Well, sure I'm angry," I say. "I have good reason to be angry. I love somebody who has no capability of returning love. Can my broken heart be healed?"

She looks at me very sharply and says, "It isn't the broken heart you should be thinking about. It's the anger."

"Isn't healing the broken heart going to alleviate my anger?"

She smiles, with wisdom in her eyes. "If you really want to heal your broken heart, then you will deal with your anger."

"Well, that will be easy. Healing a broken heart's easy. If all I have to do is deal with my anger, I'll just say I'm angry."

Grandmother Moon looks at me with a raised eyebrow.

"Now, you know, Wolf, healing is much, much more than that. Which is why it's misunderstood. Healing is resolving. It's restoring. It's improving. It's feeling oneself. It's settle and clean. The things that enrage a person, the things that bring about anger, those things are lessons. They are painful. They are broken dreams; they are letdowns; they are passions of the broken heart and love affairs gone wrong, and all because they were constituted by unrealistic thoughts and a lack of understanding. Most people die from a broken heart. Most people grieve themselves to death from sadness and loneliness and anger. Healing is a gift. It is given to you in blue light. You'll receive your healing in the silver shimmering of the water where the full moon comes forever. It's easy to be angry. You'll find calm and peacefulness in the shimmering of the water."

"So calmness is what heals anger, Grandmother? All I have to do is just get calm and look, and this broken heart of mine will be gone?"

"Yes, I need you to look at the water," she says.

I look at the river and I see a silver shimmer. But in my heart is a blackness, a darkness that feels as if it's trying to take my breath away. I want to go there. It would be so easy to go there. But I remember her words. The soft silver shimmer intensifies the blue of the river, and I feel a warm, gentle tranquility come over me. I look back at Grandmother.

"What is the blackness, Grandmother, that comes from me? Is it anger?"

Grandmother looks out at the river. "It is from the depth of darkness, the depth of ignorance and a lack of energy that illness emerges—that blackness, that emptiness, that ignorance I have known for all my existence. From the spiral of the whiteness of the moon to the gold of the moon to the darkness of the moon and the fullness of the moon. I have seen that. And with the ebb and flow of life, the water comes and washes it all away."

I put my hands behind my head and lean back on the rock. It is so wonderful to look at Grandmother's face and feel the calmness of my heart. It's quite magical that all I have to do is let go and remember the silver shimmering. "What is the silver shimmer, Grandmother?"

She says, with laughter in her voice, "Well, is it anger, Granddaughter?"

"No, it's not anger," I say. "Grandmother, I feel a feeling that I've never felt before. It is really new to me."

"Well, what does it feel like?"

"It's round. It's spiraling. It's very complex, Grandmother. I want to say it's happy, but it's bigger than that."

I feel her soft hand touch mine. "It is complex, Granddaughter. But it is yours—yours to keep forever. The magic of the shimmer on the water is joy."

I decide to build a fire and sit for the rest of the night, thinking about the words I have heard. As I look at a circle of stones to my left, teeny frogs appear. Each stone has a frog sitting on top of it, and each frog has a smile on its face. The first frog says, "I am solving. I am the frog of how to solve." The next frog says, "I am curing. I am the frog of curing." The next stone's frog says, "I am restoring. I am the frog of restoring." The next frog says, "I am improving!" The next one, "I am feeling oneself." The next frog says, "I am settle!" The last frog says, "I am clean," and a soft rain begins to fall over me. Each frog begins to sing, and I hear a symphony in their little sounds.

I turn, but she has disappeared into the mist of the river. I can hear a rippling, voices on the rocks. I turn back and there is a circle on the ground. I hear Grandmother's voice in the songs of the river, the trickling of the water over the stones.

I sit here thinking of the words I hear in the frogs' songs—clearing and cleansing, thinking of the love I still feel, thinking of the promises that had been made to me.

"Well, what would you wish—what would you want to wish for—if you only had one wish?" I hear a deep, familiar voice from behind me. Oh, I don't even have to turn around. I know I would be looking into those Dark Eyes. "What would you wish for, Wolf!"

For a moment my mind is filled with a journey along the rolling river that wove its way through the gentle mountains with boulder and rock shores and flint that lined the creek, for the water was pure and clear. "Oh ho, I would wish for those days. The days of my youth, the youth of everybody. I would wish for those days, the days when I learned to fall in love, the days when I learned what love is."

"Well, in your complicated way of looking at things, Wolf, I'm sure you'll recognize it and rationalize it out to be an emotion. I'm sure you'll say that love is simply a feeling that comes and goes. You're angry with *me* for making promises. I told you I would never promise anything and you pushed me. You asked me to promise. You said 'Promise me.' Your fear was so deep that it made a spiraling pit that you fell into."

It is that deep, dark emptiness in his voice that makes me turn around, because it is a challenge to stand once more in the presence of those Dark Eyes and look into the depth of emptiness. There stands in front of me one who cannot love.

"Heh, heh," he laughs. "I can not love? How can you be so vicious and cruel? Your anger cuts into my heart. Is it the promise that you pushed me to make, or is it your anger that eats your heart?"

Looking at him, I see one who cannot commit and stay, one who is illusive. There are strong features in his beveled face, a dark beard, long hair braided thick and strong, a massive thickness in his shoulders and arms, beveled stomach, thin waist, strong thighs, and muscled calves. The perfectly built two-legged male, the stamina of the elk. The moon glistens in his raven hair. The night dances in his eyes.

"I have learned to beware of the darkness, I have learned to watch for the void in your eyes." I take a deep breath.

"I'm sure you have," he replies. "You have figured it all out. You have figured out illusiveness. Have you been able to catch me? Have you been able to do the moon dance and leap from one stone to the next down the river, and chase me into the night? Have you been able to remain young forever? Will you dance with me in the moonlight, tonight, forever?" His laughter rings out and echoes off the walls of the canyon that lines the river where we are standing.

"There isn't any staying with you forever," I reply. "I have come to an understanding that there is no night in you. Yes, I've learned what illusiveness is. It is myself. It is in my passion and anger that I give you power. I have no desire to give up my life, drop my head and lose my pride."

"I never asked you to," he says.

"I have walked along the river. I have come here once again to face my own inadequacies. It was my passion for you that brought me to my knees."

He looks away from me.

"And I have come here to mend my broken heart," I say, "my grandmother, a dear one, has reminded me that it is anger that has brought me to my knees. It is sadness that has brought me down to this place where I am annoyed, where I become belligerent and violent."

"Look out, look out for him," goes through my mind.

"I sat within her healing circle. In healing, the answers came to me," I say.

His laughter is familiar as he walks closer to me. "Dare you dance in the moonlight tonight?" he asks. "Dare you dance the moon dance?" He leans forward. "Reach out and touch my hand."

In his hand he has a small bunch of dark blue berries. He rubs them together with his other hand, turning one hand blue and placing it on his chest. "It is the hand print of eternity. It is the blue of the river that flows in the moonlight. It is the blue of the sky. It is life," he says. "Dance with me in the moonlight. Stay with me and there won't be any need for healing."

Oh, I feel myself weaving, becoming faint and disappearing, going within my yearning—the crush of long ago—my heart losing its air, losing its energy, my lungs collapsing. As he opens the other hand, a swirling blue smoke encompasses me. It is my breath. Before me is the blackness, the depth of loneliness and emptiness. It could be any disease—call it what you may—emptiness is at bay, standing, waiting for me. It is simply a step through. Transformation. Transform yourself into smoke. Be of the clouds.

Night has fallen. The deep shades of blue are reflected on the water in the moonlight. Silver and blue are all I see. I spin, I swirl. The blackness engulfs me. The thick gom, gooey void is now my battlefield. Whatever it is—disease, broken heart, emotional distress, anger, out of control—this is now my struggle. It chokes, it limits, it confuses me. I stay steady in silver. I breathe narrow and soft. It is choking me with its desire to contain and control. I can feel the passion, I can feel the rage. I can feel the need— "Hold me, embrace me, keep me . . ."

"No!" I say. Inside, deep inside, I push away. There is no getting away from the darkness.

"Stay! Become!"

I delve deeper into the void, searching for immortality, youth, success, spontaneity. I grab for it.

"BE CAREFUL! BE CAREFUL!" he says. "I'm dangerous! Hold me gently. You'll be marked and never be able to let go."

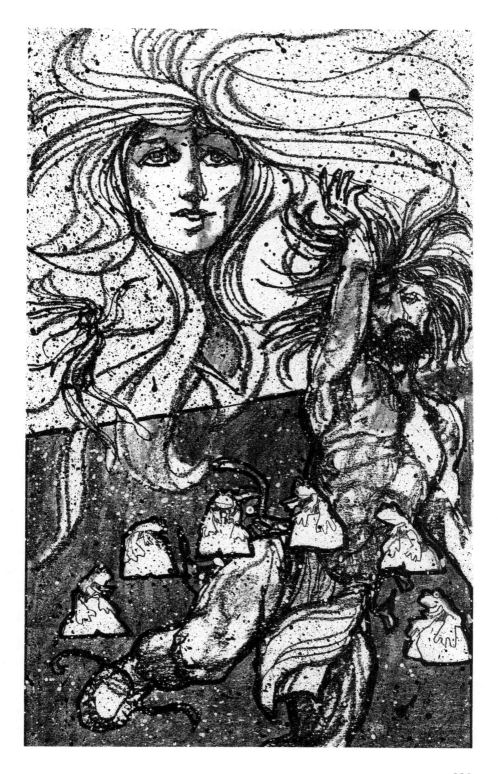

I have embraced broken hearts, illness, insanity, anger, and rage. I have it all now in my hands. It takes all my strength. The wolf energy rages through my body; my hands are strengthened. "Hold on for just a few more moments," I think.

A fierceness, a whirlwind spins me around. I am spinning and twisting. No plans, no organization, just *now*. Holding on.

"Remember, I'm dangerous," the soft, deep familiar voice echoes.

"Danger is nothing to me," I say. I see an opening in the sky. There is color, peace, tranquility, and transformation. "It has begun."

I hear the shrieks, screams, and moans of many others, agonizing over eternal youth, wishing to dye their hair and paint their nails, trying to hold on. Trying to hold on to the cheapness of life, to buy it with a few dollars, to gain it with material things. The beauty and the magnificence of the mountains and the moonlight remain my path, the quiet of the river that rolls on through the night, the gentleness of the swooping, soft hillsides— life, stars, beyond.

"Hold on," I think. "Ride it out its full eight seconds. Give it the best ride there is. It is the ride of life. Let loose not, lest ye die. Many cultures and beliefs spiral through my head. How could people come to a land and totally dominate it with disrespect?

"I must hold on, Wolf, I must hold on," I tell myself.

The darkness increases. The spiraling, the spinning, the whirlwind, the noise grows louder in my mind, but the blue smoke comforts me. From the moon shines a blue light. I begin to walk on that light. I emerge from the choking and the dying, from the bitterness and anger. I feel a gentleness, like a soft breeze as I walk the path towards the moon, leaving behind the dangerous, the lack of respect, the greed, and the envy, the Dark Eyes. I walk beyond on the moonbeam. Days and days and days I walk, remembering his deep voice, his dark eyes, the promises. I let go.

Before me I can see the glistening and the sparkling of the rainbow on the river. Following the moon path I walk into a valley. I stand there. The land is quiet. Eagles are large; deer are plentiful, as are the hawks, bears, and horses. Before me I see the healing circle. The stones are big. There are four stones in the circle and a weasel stands in the center.

"Yeah. Yeah, you've got it all together now, don't you?" he says. "You've received your healing, right? Right? Listen to these words—cure. Have you been cured? Settle. Are you all settled? How about belligerent and violent?" His small nose twitches. His beady little eyes stare at me. "Have you really, Wolf, found the answers? Maybe you had better cry out for your Grandmother Moon again."

The weasel runs off, but stops after a few steps and says, "You know the story of a weasel, don't you?" He licks his lips. "I eat the eggs. That's my purpose. To destroy life. I sneak, I wiggle, and I slither. I'm smarter than the snake, you know?" he licks his lips again.

I hear the coyotes baying in the background. I feel the loneliness in my heart.

Maybe I have betrayed those Dark Eyes. Maybe I didn't hear what he was saying at all. Maybe it was the passion and the violence. Maybe it was my addiction to anger.

In front of me I see a fire. A dancer emerges from it—a beautiful, silver dancer. She spins and swirls around the fire. The silver and the gold of the fire become two rings and a united force. The fire is now silver and gold. She dances, hair flowing in the breeze. Her spirit becomes mine.

"Dance with me, Wolf. The Dance of the Moon."

The dancer and I begin to move around the fire. Evening comes, then early night with a soft, blue sky. Stars, silver points of light, are dancing all around me. The blue smoke filters across the ground and I feel the arms of Dark Eyes around me. We dance together in perfect harmony.

"Who promises, he says, "me or you? What is it that you fear? Could it be your anger that opens the door to your fear? You have no Acceptance, you cannot let go."

Fiercely, we dance together. At last, the passion becomes quiet and our hearts beat as one. I sway with the wind. As one we walk each step in the dance. We have danced together for so long, each step across those rocks. He leaps, I leap. Each rock we leap—one after another, I follow him down the river. Quickly, one stone after another. He jumps to the side, and I jump to the side. He floats on the wave, and I float on the wave. We move together as one all night, into the sunrise.

I wake with the sun on my face. The warm memories of the healing circle curing, solving, restoring, settling, and cleansing. I can remember the silver stars glistening in the night.

I hear the soft sounds of the stars calling me back.

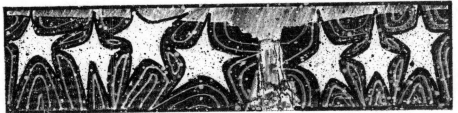

The Emotional Teachings of Anger

Build a mini-wheel for Anger by placing Anger in the center. In the spirit place Passionate; in the feelings place Annoyed; in the totality place Violent; and in the concept of Anger place Belligerent.

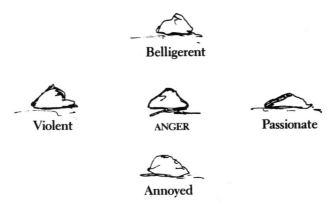

Belligerent

Violent ANGER **Passionate**

Annoyed

Make a list of your passions, such as rage, rampage, wrath, lust, idolizing, yearning, love, crush.

> *Example: rage. You met someone that you want to have a relationship with, and that person rejects you. You cannot handle the rejection, and retaliate with physical violence.*

Under feelings, list the things that annoy you, such as reacting, challenges, competition, proving.

> *Example: reacting. A person you want to have a relationship with dates you twice, and then tells you that he or she doesn't want to see you anymore. You say you never wanted to go out with him or her anyway.*

Under totality, list your violent totality of anger, such as hateful, spiteful, explosive, crafty, self-destructive, suicidal or homicidal impulses.

> *Example: suicidal. After you've been rejected by the person who does not want to date you again, you decide to lock yourself in your bathroom and slash your wrists.*

Under concept, list your belligerence, such as ballistic, intolerant, destructive, selfish, stubborn, despondent.

Example: selfish. You constantly think of the person and having another date, even though the person has terminated the relationship. You continue to think of yourself and the person together.

As I mentioned before, when you are studying your mini-wheel, it is a good idea to go to your dictionary and thesaurus to look up the definitions of these words. It may be an eye-opener to you. Be sure you journal your feelings about what you have read. Ask yourself, when you study the emotion of Anger, "How do I apply these words in my life? Where do I see these actions?"

If you don't feel this exercise can work for you, I would suggest anger-management counseling. If you experience violent or suicidal behaviors, I recommend that you seek out a shaman who works in psychiatry on anger management.

Ceremony of the Moon

Tools: *Rocks—the number can vary. You'll need not less than 25 and possibly as many as 100. I recommend that they be equal in value to the subject matter you are going to work with—small, medium, and large; paint, washable and water soluble; paintbrush; paint in the seven colors—red, orange, yellow, green, blue, purple, and burgundy; smudge bowl, sweet grass and sage; a stick that is two feet (.6m) tall; a strip of red cloth one inch wide by 24 inches (2.5 × 60cm) long; your spirit journal and pen.*

You'll need a quiet place where you will be undisturbed, and where you can build a circle of rocks. The ceremony can be done inside or outside, and remember you can do the ceremony by simply visualizing it in your mind.

The Ceremony of the Moon, a healing circle, starts when you have chosen the proper place to hold the ceremony. The healing circle is built from stones that are connected to your Medicine and Lesson words. The circle is a place in which you go to work with the lessons that you are achieving.

The healing circle is one in which you stand at least 15 minutes a day working with the seven Lesson Words of the South. These words are:

Clarity—red
Poise—orange
Discipline—yellow
Account—green
Fact—blue
Sense—purple
Complete—burgundy.

When you need to work with a lesson to understand it or to gather knowledge from it, you apply your Medicine Words from the South, which are:

Strength—red
Success—orange
Vision—yellow
Beauty—green
Healing—blue
Power—purple
Great—burgundy.

1. When you build a healing circle, you start by honoring the space where the circle sits. You do this by lighting the sweet grass and sage and letting the smoke drift over the place where the circle will sit. Use your hands to work the smoke completely over the area.

The healing circle is a shamanic place that allows you to be in both the physical and spiritual worlds. You can go to your healing circle any time of the day or night and any time of the month or year to study, to dismiss, or to bring about Strength. It's a good idea to remember that one of the qualities of shamanism is being in two places at one time. Even if you are limited to the physical plane, you can move within the spirit world, thereby connecting these two planes together.

The healing circle will be a circle of stones that you bring forth by connecting one stone to each lesson or medicine that you understand, have learned, or apply.

2. After you have smudged, place the stick as the center point if you're outside, digging in the ground. If you're inside, you can put the stick in the center of the room in any container that you can fill with dirt to hold the stick upright. Then tie the red flag to the stick.

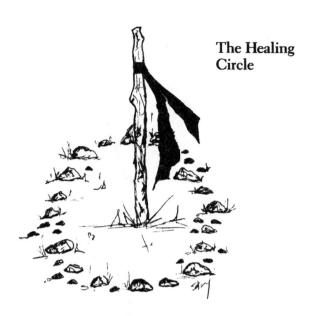

The Healing Circle

3. You then determine the direction of the East. You can find it by looking at where the sun rises at dawn. Mark that direction with an unpainted stone; it will represent the beginning of your healing circle. You can place the stone as far away from the center stick as you have room. The size of the circle will be determined by the size and number of stones used. But, remember that a healing circle need only be one stone placed next to the direction stone (East) because the stone itself is a circle.

4. When you are standing in the East at the direction stone, looking at the flag and the center point, your lessons will go on the left-hand side. You will place them around in an arc to the point where you are facing the direction stone. When you are standing at the direction stone and looking at the flag, your Medicine Rocks will start where your Lesson Rocks end. Place the Medicine Rocks in an arc on the right side of the circle.

5. Sit at your direction stone (East) with your journal and pen. Make a list of your lessons that are within Clarity. Apply your emotional acceptance to that Lesson Rock by listing where you have been accepting of the lesson of Clarity.

> ***Example:*** *It is clear to me that human life has an end point, that all humans die. It was a lesson of Clarity that I learned as a child when I lost a loved one. When I lost the next loved one, I applied Acceptance to death through my Clarity that all humans die.*

List as many lessons of Clarity with the emotion of Acceptance in answer to them as you can.

6. Now list your medicine of Strength that enabled you to accept the lesson.

Example: Death was hard to comprehend the first time a loved one died. The second time I experienced death was when I saw one of my cats run over by a car. Years passed, and then I experienced the death of a sister. I understood that humans, animals, and all things die. From this knowing came the Strength to endure my sister's death. If I must experience another death, I will use my medicine of Strength to give me support.

7. When you have listed as many Strengths as you can, take one rock for each lesson of Clarity and one rock for each medicine of Strength. You will paint a dot on your Lesson Rock in the appropriate color for the lesson, and you will paint a star on your Medicine Rock in the appropriate color for the medicine. You will place each Lesson Rock to the left of the direction stone (East) and each Medicine Rock to the right, moving clockwise, starting equally across from the direction stone.

You will continue placing stones for each lesson and for each medicine.

8. You have applied Acceptance to the lesson of Clarity. Now apply:
Disgust to the lesson of Poise;
Happy to the lesson of Discipline;
Sad to the lesson of Account;
Anger to the lesson of Fact;
Fear to the lesson of Sense;
Joy to the lesson of Complete.

Be sure that when you are listing your lessons you speak of each one of your emotions.

Example: Disgust applied to Poise. If you are overweight, but are out enjoying yourself shopping in a mall, and someone makes fun of your obesity, this is disgusting. To overcome Disgust, obtain the lesson of Poise by standing firm in what is so—that in fact you are obese—but to an obese person, skinny could be disgusting.

Example: Happy applied to Discipline. You do your prayer ties each day, offering one prayer to Great Spirit, four prayers to honor each direction, and seven prayers to honor the medicines/lessons. You tie your prayer ties on your line each day, and this relationship brings you happiness. This is applying Happy to Discipline.

Example: Sad applied to Account. *You bring home your paycheck, you enter the amount into your budget, and you are saddened that you don't have enough money to obtain your goals. This is applying Sad to Account. It is extremely important to recognize your sadness in your daily account of life.*

Example: Anger applied to Fact. *You're living your life thinking that your father was deceased when you were born, and then it turns out that you have no father because you were a product of rape. This produces extreme anger towards your father. This is applying Anger to Fact.*

Example: Fear applied to Sense. *You are walking home at night after attending a sports event, and you sense someone looking at you. You feel strongly that you are being followed. You know that you have two blocks to go before reaching your house. You have to choose between going straight home or taking a longer route. Because your sense of being watched becomes stronger, you decide to go the long way home. You awaken the next morning to learn that there was a killing on the street you would have taken if you had gone straight home. This is applying Fear to Sense.*

Example: Joy applied to Complete. *A personal example of this is achieving this book. When a book is complete, it is my joy knowing that these words are here for you to read. This is Joy applied to Complete.*

As you have applied your emotions to your lessons, you have laid a rock in the circle for each lesson. As you have applied your medicines to the lessons, you do the same. You may choose to work with only one lesson and lay only one stone. That could be with any one of the seven lessons/medicines you wish. You could have many lessons/medicines in one day. For each lesson make sure you connect your emotions, and also place a stone on the medicine side of the circle. Your healing circle is complete when you have sat with the direction stone and faced your pole with the red flag.

During the period of time that you are working with your healing circle, I recommend that you visit it once a day to look at the pole and see that you are bringing about a success in healing.

9. When you feel you are done with the healing circle, cleanse the stones by washing the paint off—with running water outdoors with a garden hose or in the sink with fast-running water. Then place the stones back where you found them and let the energy from the circle go.

Remove the stick from the center. Remove the flag, placing the stick back where you found it. Take the red flag and cut it into one-inch (2.5cm) squares, and make prayer ties for the memory of the healing circle. Place these prayers on the line with your others.

10. If there is a day when you don't have a broken heart or a bad dream or an unpleasant experience, when there is no Anger, Disgust, Fear, or Sadness, then it is a good day. It is a wonderful day because you will be working with your Strength and Success. You will have your mind on your Vision, and your Beauty in your heart. You will be walking with the constant transformation of the cycle and the circle of sacred power that you have within yourself, which gives you your Greatness. You can stand tall, look into the sky and say "Thank you, Grandmother and Grandfather, for I had a good day. I know the lesson of Clarity, I have my Poise, my Discipline is that I am here with you. I Account for the things in my life I know to be Fact. It makes Sense and I am Complete."

Aho.

Spirit Shirt Vision of the Frog

Find a quiet place where you can go to have your vision, where you won't be interrupted. Sit, close your eyes, and breathe in and out four times. Breathe in and out, and relax. Let your mind just be free. Before you, you'll see a silver path, a path that is a moonbeam. This moonbeam lights up a path along a river and you can see the shimmer on the river. You look up the moonbeam, and it takes you to the sky. You look up, and there is a full moon, Grandmother Moon. You look at her and you can see your symbol for the Dance of the Moon. Remember this symbol and bring it back to your spirit journal. Draw the symbol. Make a green circle with a blue circle just inside it and place the symbol inside. Now transfer the symbol to your spirit shirt.

Medicine Rocks

To have a medicine rock is to have a whole new arena of medicine that comes from the mineral world. The medicine rock has a grounding energy with which it balances weak energy. There is a soothing and smoothing, as the energy of the mineral meshes with the energy of the minerals in your body. It brings forth and expands; it widens; it opens; it makes strong. As it strengthens your energy, it uplifts and stabilizes you. It helps you to focus.

Medicine rocks are chosen by the kind of rock they are. All rocks are medicine rocks; all rocks have medicine. But different kinds of rocks have different uses. Semi-precious rocks are chosen strictly for their color. Granites, agates, and plain mud or dirt rocks are good to paint and place vision symbols on. Then there are the "wish stones," which have a white circle all the way around them and are often found along the water,

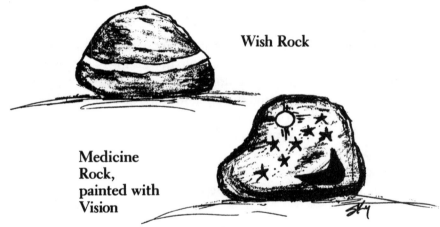

Wish Rock

Medicine Rock, painted with Vision

especially beside the ocean. There is one called the sacred holy rock—the rock of vision—that has a hole in it; you can look all the way through it. This rock is used for focusing and centering. You can also use it for looking into the spirit world. You do that by looking through the rock, letting your mind relax, and seeing what you see. The holy rock is one of the most sought after rocks. You should have only one of them. If you covet a bunch of holy rocks, you will take someone else's stone. These rocks have been made by thousands of years of water drops falling in one spot, causing the hole to open up, and they are rare.

When you decide that you are going to carry a stone that is painted or has a vision symbol on it, select the rock and cleanse it with saltwater and fresh running water. Then place it on top of a crystal. Crystals are charging stones, and their energy expands the balance of solid rock. Then paint the rock with any medicine symbol that you have received through the vision that comes from the rock. Then it becomes a medicine rock to treat whatever issue you selected it for.

It is a good thing to paint medicine rocks with the symbols from your vision shirt. You can carry them in your pouches, or you can wear them, making jewelry from them. You can place your spirit animals or totems on them. You carry your medicine rock around with you to draw energy from it, to focus you, and to help you feel comfortable. One of the wonderful things about a medicine rock is that when you carry it, you are never alone, for you have the strength, the teachings, and the knowledge that comes from the stone itself—its type, its character, its color, as well as the power from the symbols you have drawn on it.

Very pale blue stones—ones that are soft blue, like aquamarine and the blue crystals—are water connections. You can use them to connect with water, and you can cleanse your spirit by seeing the stone become water rushing over you.

Whether you carry the rock in your pocket or wear it on your body, a medicine rock must have its own pouch. To make a medicine pouch, take a piece of cloth, pull it up over the stone and tie it around the top with a red string. Circle the string around the top four times and then make a loop so you can wear the pouch around your neck. You can place the rock in a bigger medicine bag, if you want, or carry it inside something else; but always wrap it up in its own pouch.

When opening the pouch, you need to smudge. Run the rock through the smudge four times and set yourself in balance.

There are many types of medicine rocks and many ways of working with them. This small amount of information for bringing forth a medicine rock will get you started.

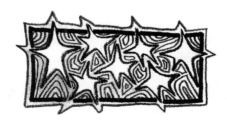

The Process of the Lesson of Fact

Fact is the lesson needed to obtain your medicine of healing. There are five steps to this process of fact.

1. Actuality. The emotion of Acceptance is the feeling of actuality, knowing that what you believe is.

> *Example: There is a sun in the sky, whether you see it or not. Knowing there will be light in the sky is your Acceptance of actuality, bringing about a fact.*

2. Details. The details of a fact will have the emotion of Disgust within them. Details are often hard to grasp and take a lot of understanding.

> *Example: The sun is behind the clouds and you haven't seen it for fourteen days. You remember the beauty of a clear day, but all you have is a cloudy gray day. This brings about Disgust to you because you want a clear day. The details of clouds get old, and you want to see the face of the sun.*

3. Experience. Within experience is the knowing of the past. You can and do remember times before and you apply them to your life. The application has within it the emotion of Happy.

> *Example: Though it is cloudy, I remember many clear days of sunshine in my life and it brings a smile to my heart (mind).*

4. Point. Within the point will be the emotion of Sad. But all in all, the point is fact.

> *Example: There is a sun, but clouds cover it, and I have a cloudy day, which saddens me because I like the clear sunshine. But there is a sun and tomorrow it will shine if there are no clouds.*

5. Reality. Within reality is the truth. You get to the point and understand that in life there will be times that are just the way they are, and you can't change them. In reality you experience the emotions of Anger, Fear, and Joy.

Example: I don't want a cloudy day (anger). I didn't think I could be happy or even want to get up, because I can't see the sun (fear). I remember the sun and its warmth. I will look forward to a sunny day because it is my hope. The sun is there and that gives me great joy.

Healing Medicine

Healing is simply a cycle. It is a reaching out, and Healing medicine is Strength in movement. It is the lesson of Discipline and Patience. It is the lesson of Clarity and Purpose. It brings about a transformation of movement that takes you from one place to the next. Healing Medicine is application and moving on. It is the Facts that are at hand, things that have happened and things that will happen. If it is fullness, richness, and wellness that you wish, then that will be your Healing. If it is to learn a lesson and get it right, then that is your Healing. Healing is a word of action. It is a word that takes place in Fact.

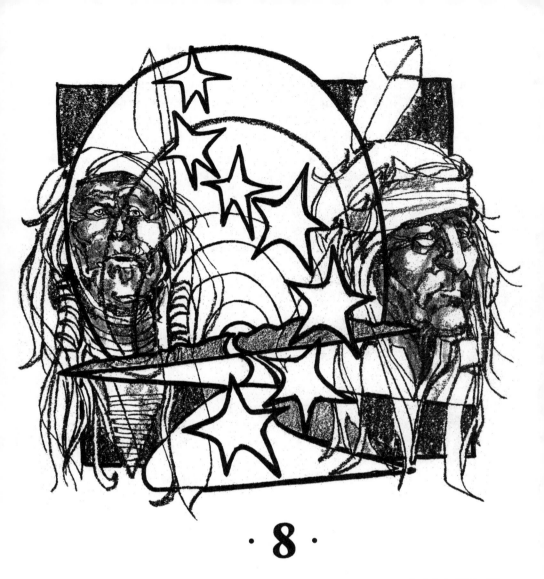

· 8 ·

THE DANCE OF THE STARS

Softly I breathe. Softly the wind blows. I feel feminine energy all around me, soft lavenders, soft purples. Softly they blow. I breathe and I relax. It's nighttime, it's dark, and I'm sitting in a circle of pines within a medicine wheel. It is quiet after the students have gone. The candles twinkle in the night—yellows, reds, whites, and others. I rattle softly, and the sounds speak in my mind—they are the voices of the stars. The little tiny grains of rock rattle back and forth; the clicking, the sounds—I hear them—

swishing sounds. I feel the energy of the ocean around me. I feel power building in the rattle.

Before me I see the ocean. I am within the ocean, a quietness as I walk along. And there, in front of me, a whale is moving towards me with grace. I am so small. It is so large. Its mouth becomes that of a cave. I go in. Inside I feel a coldness, a darkness and an emptiness. Fear comes to me. I feel this shock! I am alarmed! I want to turn and run, but I am overcome by amazement. I am inside a whale! I walk on, still hearing the rattling sound that connects me to earth. The whale is really huge. Before me stands a woman with black hair. She is dressed all in black, except for one side of her face, which is painted white. She is large but sleek. Her clothing is like tight rubber. I feel anxiety move across me. Sometimes I have a coward energy inside. I wish to run.

"No, stand still, Wolf. I have things to say to you, for you are in the breath itself. Within the whale you must face your panic. On Earth we know the word as phobia. On Earth we are all afraid. The alarm you felt was warning you to turn back, but you stepped on. There are lessons to learn about fear before you can dance on the stars and move within Greatness. You must understand in order to revere. You must understand in order to respect. When you hold within you the medicine of Power, you have a gift—the ability, the strength, and the energy to move on."

I see now she is wearing a necklace of whale teeth. There are four of them and they are immense—one of them is nine inches by at least four. She is strong and powerful; her eyes are deep.

"If you wish to return and walk as a two-legged and carry with you your Power, you must face your fear NOW."

I feel myself fall backwards. I am underwater. I spin, end over end, moving backwards. I find myself lying in the forest with my head on a log. I have a headache and I am dizzy. It is dark, and cold. All around me I can see red—there are red dots; there are red eyes. I see a figure before me that is neither male nor female, but it is in human form with hooves for feet. On its hands are long fingernails. Its head has horns that come up and curl like those of a ram. Its eyes are a piercing red. Its breath is foul and ugly.

"Your childhood is in your face," the creature hisses. "It is within each of us to create a devil. It is within each of us to create the boogeyman."

My heart is pounding. It sounds like a drum. I look through the creature but it's still there. To its side there are others. Their teeth are those of fierce bears and mountain lions and wolves. Their faces are repulsive. I can hear the words of the whale woman—"revere" and "respect." But my cowardliness! The way I want to run! Each one of these spirits becomes a tombstone.

144

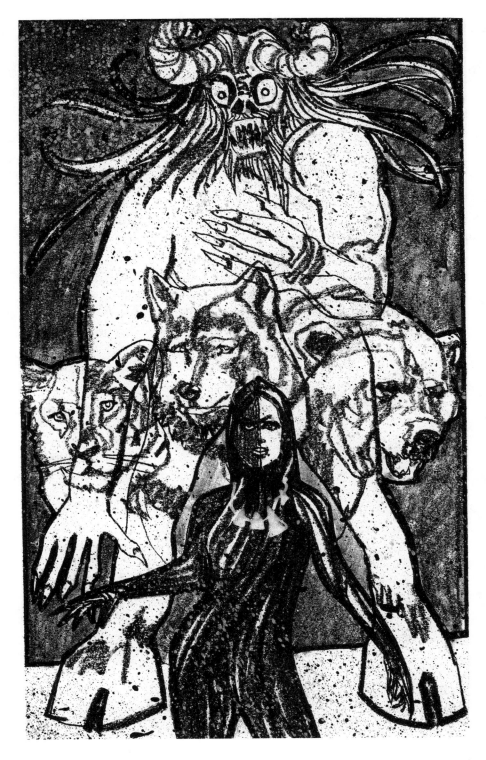

I stand in a graveyard, empty and cold. On one side of me is a tombstone with the name of my father and in front of me is a grave marked "Nobody." Around me are the tombstones of my husband, my children, my friends. I can hear the owl. It is calling for me, hooting, "Wolf." I take a deep breath and relax. I try to draw on my abilities. I try to stand solid in my Strength, but my energy is fading. I can hear the waves of water inside the whale's stomach. I try to find some tranquility, but the owl keeps calling my name. Suddenly, beside me on a tree, lands a white owl. It takes the form of the most beautiful woman. Her hair is flowing and full. She is definitely White Owl Woman. She speaks to me with grace and peace.

"You have your Strength, Wolf. You must listen to your own phobias. You must listen to your own panic. One of the things you must know is that for all the darkness and evil that mankind has brought forth to wrench their souls, for all the dismay, amazement, and alarm—they are the torchbearers of Truth within Power. For you to walk within your wholeness of Power, and to carry it as a teacher, you must know you have a gift. I have often been spoken of as the Omen of Death. The hour of death is now."

A black horse runs past me, fierce and beautiful. It is superb and impeccable, imperial and flawless. It stops, throws its head up, and shakes its mane out full. Then it arches its tail and gallops into the wind. The night becomes a deeper shade of purple.

"Did you see that, Wolf?"

I look at the woman and ask her name. "I'm White Owl Woman. Listen to me. Everyone dies, within both worlds. Within time you must descend. Within time you will step forth into a place beyond, where ancestors and elders live, where peace comes into your heart. You must understand it is a gift of life to die."

She smiles, and her face is radiant. I see past her round yellow eyes into deep blue human eyes. Her face is soft and pink, her hair is silver. I recognize her as a good friend of mine, a student who has sat with me. I recognize her willowy form as a grace in understanding the gift of life, which is death.

"Sit with me, Wolf, here in the woods, and listen in the quiet wet of the night. Listen to me carefully when I speak and let your panic drip into the ground. Let go of your dismay. Understand that death is simply that silver door there."

She points. It is an awesome sight—this shimmer of color glittering in the night, a doorway to the brightest white I have ever seen. Suddenly the door opens and for a moment the light takes my sight away. Out come dancers, all colors. Winged ones and four-legged, they dance, they sing.

146

Around the circle they go, prancing and dancing the moon and the rose. Dancing the Earth. And there is Yellow Bird. Beyond that I see my relatives—aunties and uncles, grandmothers.

"Join them, Wolf. Soon you will. For this opportunity that we bring about—alarm and amazement—we should have reverence and respect. I am the Grandmother of Fear. You see, it is often said that when the White Owl calls, it is time to leave. I have come to you as a sister. White Wolf Woman, look within yourself and listen. Draw from your strength of the wolf. Know that you walk in the North, and it is the mind that is the corridor that leads to the soul. Know that the rainbow is simply a step across from one place to the other, and that the North oversees the children. In legends, both of us are spoken of as very scary, and there are even those who say the owl is the most evil of all. They say that I can put curses on you, that I am a witch, that I have long black fingernails—when they are simply my talons.

"Looking back on the Earth now, we see that our homes are becoming scarce and people want to do away with us out of their own phobias. Cut down the trees and destroy the homes of the owls. Even Native Americans shriek and worry over an owl feather. Wolf, I speak to you about anxiety and dismay. I hope that all will open up their hearts to Power and understand their abilities. How can they reach their life's expectations when they cannot hear Great Spirit, Grandmother, Grandfather?"

Eee—I can hear a storm building behind her—thunder and a small flick of lightning. She hoots and says, "Maybe the most evil of all shall appear. Have you revered Satan itself?"

Uh, that feeling is back. Looking out into the darkness, I know there is something there that is going to get me! She raises her arm and fans me with the softness of her feathers. My heart races. But I can see the breath within the Whale Woman. I remember her softness, her firmness, and how vast the whale is. I am prepared to meet evil.

White Owl Woman laughs and says, "It is not evil that you will meet in human form, ever. It is always fear. What we know to be evil are simply acts of fear and anger. We put energy into our lives to bring our fear into manifested form."

She places before me a silver pouch. "Open this pouch, Wolf, and you will find the path to the Great Waterfall. Then you will be with your Grandmother and Grandfather Wolf once more and hear their words of wisdom. How do you feel?"

I take a deep breath as I look down at the silver pouch that lies on the ground. "I feel solid."

I look past her and there stands a cloaked, black spirit, glaring at me, its eyes dull and red and cold. I glance back at the silver pouch and forget what I have seen. It is just a figment of my imagination.

"Ah," she says, "you're getting it now. Everything—anxiety, panic, alarm—we have those feelings for reasons. They are there to warn us, to bring about respect."

I look down, and in my hand is the silver pouch.

"Open the pouch," she says.

I open the pouch and let it go. Out before me run stars—millions and millions and millions of stars—trillions of them—all colors. And among them I can see the purest and prettiest purple. It is a color I shall never forget. As they run I can see they are all, all colors, all spirit, all existence. They make a beautiful road, a path of twinkling and glittering stars.

"Dance the star dance. Dance the dance of the stars, Wolf, and follow them beyond. There are so many levels of spirit. So many levels of understanding. Dance beyond where you are now and move to a deeper level within your life."

I follow the stars to what seems higher in the sky than where I was. I walk on points of light. I come to a place of quiet in the night where I can sit on the stars and still watch them. The stars are everywhere. They shimmer and glisten. I can hear them singing. Their sounds are soft, twinkling, female sounds—high notes, precious notes. Before me a spirit emerges, a spirit of deep, rich purple—pale purples, soft lavender. The wind blows through this spirit; it is transparent. Its hair is shimmering silvery purple, lavender. Stars are its fingertips and toes. Stars are its eyes and the tips of its hair. It moves in a spiraling, swaying motion when it walks. It glides on the star path. It comes closer and closer to me, until finally it sits cross-legged in front of me.

"I am a Star Being, Star Person, Star." As it sits there it sways from side to side. It is fluid motion. Its features and body are of human shape, but it is all star, transparent.

"I give to you now, Wolf, something that you need." It holds its hand out and in its palm it has a beautiful star-shaped amethyst. "This is a gift, the gift of Power, which is what Power is. Power is your gift. I give you the amethyst so that you are careful not to overuse your Power. In this star I give you ability. The ability is your Strength. Your energy is here, Wolf. Hold out your hand."

I hold out my hand and it places the star in it. The star energy sways back and forth. "You now have your power. It is important to learn, when you have your Power, that your lessons are all in Balance. That you have Clarity and Poise, that there be Discipline, that you account the Facts and you have your Power. And now, there before you, you'll find the path that takes you to Great and re-unites you with the teachings of your Grandmother, Grandfather Wolf."

I hear the Great Waterfall.

"Watch. Watch for the mist. Enter through the mist carefully and listen to the lessons. You will then be in the presence of the Great Waterfall of your family. Remember what you have learned. Beware of your fear. Be careful and listen, for fear is not dismay, discord, and disharmony, or ugly and evil. It is given you to ring an alarm so that you have the ability to have amazement, to revere and to respect. Wolf, you must remember respect."

I hear the soft sounds of the stars calling me back.

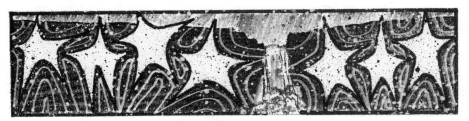

The Emotional Teachings of Fear

Build a mini-wheel by placing Fear in the center. In the spirit position is reverence; in the feelings is alarm; in totality is amazement; in concept is respect.

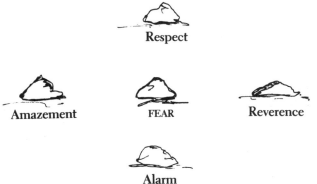

Respect

Amazement   **FEAR**   **Reverence**

Alarm

1. In your spirit journal make a list of what you have reverence for in your spirit of fear.

Example: **Mighty.** *The force of a wild storm with great amounts of wind.*
Forceful. *A forest fire out of control.*
Exhausting. *The force of a sub-zero wind in the winter that makes just walking to your car hard work. It makes you feel as if you will freeze to death quickly.*

2. Make a list of things that alarm you in your feelings of fear.

Example: **Alert.** *You have lived through many cold winters and are alert and aware that each storm is a serious condition.*
Pay attention. *You know the storm is coming and you must be ready with food, water, firewood, and warm clothes.*
Awake. *It is easy to say you are okay and have power in your home and electric heat, but you stay awake to the fact that the power could be blown out by harsh winds.*

3. Make a list of your amazement within fear.

Example: **Stop.** *You take time to listen to the weather and know when the storm will hit.*
Look. *You check outside from time to time to see if the weather is changing.*
Knowing. *You look at the temperature to see if it's going down. You listen to see if the wind has come up strongly.*

4. Make a list of the concept of respect within fear.

Example: **Remember.** *You compare today to other bad winter storm days to see how the wind and temperature compare. You respect the changes between today's storm and the others, not anticipating that the situation will necessarily be the same now.*
Alert. *You hear the wind coming up and the temperature is very low. You respect the memory of other storms and you prepare by building a fire to keep warm, or put on warmer clothes.*
Surrender. *You respect the fact that the storm is going to be bad.*

Remember, when you are working with your mini-wheel and you are working in the section of fear, that fear is not only an alarm, it is amazement, reverence, respect, dismay, anxiety, cowardice, phobias, and panic. Remember that fear was given to you so that the movement of its spirit, which is reverence, will be able to uplift you. In the feelings section, alarm tells you that something is out of balance. In the totality part of the wheel, amazement gives you the ability to back up and look, and be overwhelmed. And the concept of respect provides a healthy attitude and a healthy concern.

Aho.

Ceremony of the Stars—Wishing on a Star

Tools: *A dark night; your journal and pen; a light to see your journal; feathers that have the ends wrapped in purple—one for each wish you want to make; and a tree to tie the feathers to.*

The Ceremony of the Stars is done at night, some time after dark. It needs to be very dark, and you need to be where you can see the stars. Get away from city lights to where the stars are clear, where you can sit with a tree or trees and still see the sky. Take your journal with you, so you can do a lot of communicating with yourself about wishing and power.

In the Ceremony of the Stars you are confronted with Power. Power is a gift—one of ability, Strength, and energy. So it is important that you learn, when you make a wish, to know that you have that wish already, within yourself and fully obtainable. When you make your wish, understand that there will be lessons connected with it. To have Power you must understand all seven of the lessons in the emotional part of the wheel. You will be working with the five main lessons of power, which are:

1. Fact, which brings about your Growth.
2. Account, which brings about your Balance.
3. Discipline, which brings about the Ceremony.
4. Poise, which brings about the Truth.
5. Clarity, which brings about your Wisdom

Through your wisdom you outline a situation that you want to bring about.

Example: *I wish for my life to be full and rich.*

When you make a wish, you need to break it down. You need to define each thing.

> **Example: I** = *Account. It's you.*
> **wish** *look forward to, or project what might happen, what might come to you because it is yours*
> **for my life** = *ownership of the self*
> **life** = *your experience, your totality*
> **to be** *a form of action to come about. Own it and line it out by saying: "To be, that there is work; that there are schedules, there is organization*
> **full** = *to be completely filled, total, and whole*
> **rich** = *the key word in this sentence. I define it as Strength and Success, Healing, and Power. Now you need to break down those words to yourself. What are they for you?*

If you wish to obtain something, then you know how. If you stay back in non-common sense, in make-believe, fantasy, disconnection, and not knowing, you cannot obtain.

People often wish for a new car, a boyfriend or girlfriend, a husband or wife, a new dog, a new house, a new job, but they don't break their wish down and look at what they need to do to achieve it. When we slow our minds down to achievement stages, then we become clear about our wish. This calls for the clerical work, organizing skills, and Discipline being applied. Within the ceremony, Discipline allows you to line out how you are going to take each step to get what you want. Frequently, people just want to hold their hand out and have something placed in it. That's because they separate physical reality from the spiritual movement of "All is." In a physical life you can't just hold your hand out and say you want a million dollars in it. A wish is a ceremony of Discipline, Account, Facts, Clarity, and Poise.

Next, make your wish. To make an effective wish, think about what you want and write it in your journal. Then breathe in and out seven times. Each time you breathe in, think about the wish. State the wish, and when you breathe out, see how you are going to get it. The seventh time, look at the stars in the sky and listen for their song.

The next step is to take a purple-wrapped feather from the ones you have prepared, one feather for each wish that you have made, and tie it into the tree, knowing that you have your Power. List the abilities that will enable you to obtain your wish. List the answers within your life. List the way you will benefit from the understanding of your wish. Bring these things forth from the feather as its sways in the breeze, hanging on the tree. Understand your wish totally, from what you have achieved within your Power. Give thanks for the Ceremony of the Stars. You can wish on a star at any time.

Spirit Shirt Vision of the Owl

Find a place that is quiet where you will be undisturbed. Sit with your journal and breathe in and out. Allow your eyes to close and continue breathing four times. You will be sitting next to a tree and you will feel spirit all around you as you lean up against the tree. You will feel yourself relaxing as you breathe in and out. In front of you, you will see a star, then another, and then another. You will be able to walk on those stars as if they were stairs to the sky. Then you will find yourself in the sky, standing on stars. You'll look down and see one star of a certain color. Remember that color. Then you will see your vision for the Dance of the Stars. Record it in your mind and bring it back to your journal. Draw a green circle with a purple circle inside of it and place your symbol there, in your journal. Then you are ready to paint it onto your spirit shirt. Aho.

Spirit Pouch of Power

There are many kinds of pouches. This one is called the "silver star pouch." It is made out of silver cloth, and it is a medicine pouch. You can keep it and use it any time you feel you have lost your power or become weak.

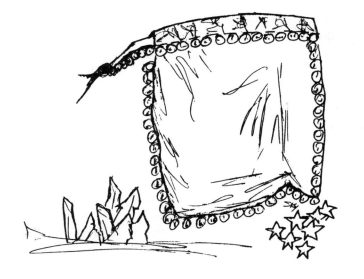

Power
Spirit
Pouch

Tools: *A half yard (.5m) of silver cloth, enough to make two 5 × 7 inch (12.5 × 17.5cm) squares; needle and silver thread; silver string to use as a drawstring; small bells or other sparkling, tinkling objects.*

Stitch the two squares together on three sides, leaving them open at the top. Then you will turn down a quarter inch of the top of the squares, and sew them in place so that a drawstring can be pulled through the top. Tie seven bells on each end of the drawstring and then stitch bells along the bottom of the pouch. You can collect all different types of little sparkling, tinkling-sounding objects to tie onto your star pouch.

Once your star pouch of power is finished, you are ready to do the ceremony that goes along with it.

Ceremony of the Silver Star Pouch

Tools: *Silver star pouch; spirit journal and pen; 7 stars, one in each of the seven colors—red, orange, yellow, green, blue, purple, burgundy. These stars can be the type found in crafts stores, or you can make them of wood or clay, or cut them from paper. They can also be made from rock, and are found in local rock shops.*

1. This ceremony may be done anytime and anywhere. Gather seven stars, one in each of the seven colors. As you make the stars or gather them, connect them to the following words. Your red one is the day you achieve your Strength. Your orange one, your Success. Yellow is your Vision. Green is your Beauty. Blue is your Healing. Purple is your Power. Burgundy is your Greatness.

Do not place any of the stars in the silver star pouch until you are sure that you can live up to the word that is connected to the color. Remember that your lessons are what separate you from the medicine. Before you have the right to carry the medicine stars in your power pouch, you must have your Clarity, you must be in Poise, have your Discipline and Account, have the Facts, make Sense, and be Complete. You can obtain the teachings of the lessons simply by sitting with the exercises in this book. Keep your stars wrapped in a cloth upon your altar until the day comes when you have learned the lessons from each star.

2. Honoring the stars. When you have journaled the meaning of each lesson and outlined how you apply it to your life in your spirit journal, then you can place the stars in your pouch and say, "I know I have my Strength because I have learned what Clarity is and listed the lesson in my journal. I have moved through the process of the lesson of Clarity, and I can apply it to my life and am ready to move in that way."

Then record your Success, if you are successful in your life. Make an entry for Vision, listing the dreams and visions you have had. List the things that are beautiful to you, and honor Healing, Power, and Greatness in the same way.

When you have journaled every word and lesson, take each star and sit with it at your altar, in your medicine wheel or in a sacred place, and light your smudge bowl. Move each star back and forth through the smoke four times for the guidance and the honoring of each direction. Then do the same with each star to represent the help of each color.

When you have honored and accepted your stars, you are ready to move on to the third movement of the ceremony.

3. Receiving the stars as yourself and placing them in the pouch. Hold the star in the air and give honor. Say a prayer, such as "Thank you, Grandmother, Grandfather, for giving me this medicine." Hold the star to your heart, hold the star up to your mouth with your hand six inches (15cm) from your mouth, and blow on it to wake it up. Then pull the air in through your mouth and take the star medicine into yourself. Finally, place the star in your silver pouch. Do this with each star. Hold the spirit of the star in your heart, in your mind. Be grateful. Hear the song of the stars in your mind. You are now able to pull the star out and use it any time you need it.

Using a Star

Remember that it is a very sacred honor to have this star. It is very sacred to have given yourself permission to say "I know what Strength is," and so on, through each color. So, holding that star out in your hand immediately allows you to know that you can apply whatever color you have—that you know how to apply that color to your life. When you are feeling weak, take out your Strength star or take out your Power star.

Take out your Greatness and apply it to your life.

Open your journal and write down what the star has to say. Go back through your journal and look at the notes that you have made about this star and apply them to your life. When you have finished, put the star back in your silver pouch, draw the cord, and place the pouch in a respectful place on your sacred altar. A sacred altar is the special area in which you keep your medicines. This could be at the base of a cross or in any other designated spot in your home. The most sacred of all altars is the medicine wheel.

You have with you now the spirit pouch of Power.

Aho.

The Process of the Lesson of Sense

Sense is having plans, goals, and dreams—and understanding your goals. When people say, "Make sense," and I say, "Make sense," it is a constitution and an outline. There is structure within Sense.

1. **For you to have Sense,** or make sense of yourself or sense of anything, you work with feelings in the spirit of the emotions—feelings of alarm, annoyance, bitterness, positive, and happy. All feelings are emotions. What makes a feeling different from an emotion is that feelings are acts and actions. Feelings are acknowledgments. They are your ability to touch your impressions to get hints, small glimpses of your consciousness. Within the lesson of Sense, list your deep feelings, how you feel about Sense.

> *Example: I feel it is very important to have an understanding of Great Spirit to make sense of life. I feel happy knowing I can do ceremony and be close to Great Spirit. I have a sense of the good life, the Red Road, when I work with my Vision and see Great Spirit's will.*

2. **Understanding within sense of yourself, life, or whatever.** Understanding is a doorway of bright light. In Star Medicine, I like to teach that understanding is your feelings. Understanding is a place where you have gathered knowledge and you know. List your understandings of Sense, what makes sense to you.

156

Encouragement: When I hear someone understand and love and make sense of life, it is an encouragement to me that I make sense. Sense is a hard thing to have and be correct. With the encouragement of others, I know the path is clear for emotional understanding.

3. Common Sense. In life we walk with our understandings.

Example: A simple thought such as appreciation of your elders, gratitude for the teachings of your grandparents, is common sense. Speaking with your family members and understanding the traditions of your family, such as birthday dinners, Thanksgiving dinner, or going to powwows—these are common sense. It is a collective group of beliefs that provide a pathway for your family.

4. Awareness. List the things you are aware of about yourself. The "awareness" part of our sense is Acceptance in a matter-of-fact way. What you are, what you look like, your weight, age, how you dress, and why these things are. When you are aware of yourself, you have a sense of yourself, your absolutes, and your likes, needs, and wants. To have a maturity within your sense of yourself, list your awarenesses, where you understand yourself and why you are the way you are. Then the sense of others will be easy. Also you will understand that Sense is the structure of experience. Within Sense is experience, which is a big part of how you make sense.

Example: You look in the mirror one day and you realize your hair is turning white. Your first thought is that you would like to dye your hair. Then you realize that maybe others have noticed the white hair and now you become panic-stricken that if you color it they'll know the truth—that you are becoming white-haired and you will seem like someone who is trying to pretend. So you stand and look in the mirror. Finally, you come to your senses and accept that you have white hair. You have witnessed other people who have white hair and they have not dyed their hair, nor have they worried about what others think. You think of these white-haired people with admiration and decide not to color your hair.

5. Brightness is the fullness of sense. To be able to understand is brightness. To be able to bring forth what you want in life is brightness. Having the ability is brightness. To have brightness, you make and can make sense of experience. Your brightness is your humor, your ability to have fun, to make other people laugh, to bring happiness and joy to others. Make a list of your brightnesses that makes sense.

Example: I get many letters full of happy comments about my books. This brings a brightness to my day. It makes writing make sense.

6. Sanity. Sane is quiet, calm, well minded, good mental health, fun and joy. Sanity is a must for sense to be so. Just plain sense of life, common sense or the sense of self. If there is no sanity there is no sense. List what sanity is to you.

Example: Sitting quietly, listening to classical music, to good country music, to rock 'n' roll, to powwow music. Reading good books, watching TV or a good movie.

Gratitude is also sanity, the ability to appreciate. List your gratitudes and appreciations.

Example: I have a nephew who studies the teaching of the medicine wheel. I am very grateful that my mother's beliefs go on.

7. Self-Esteem. Often in life we want to do something—play music, teach, bead, whatever—and, in Sense, self-esteem is needed. The sense of being able to do something calls for self-esteem. List examples of your self-esteem in your journal.

Example: When my mom passed away, she told me that she wanted my sister to carry on her talent of beading. She had a sense within her that my sis could bead and I could teach her. I felt self-esteem; I had a belief in my own beading, and I felt that I could make beading happen with my sister. I remembered what my mom had taught me, "Make sense of anything and you can do it." I did. I studied beading, remembered, and introduced my sister to it, keeping my mother's sense of the fine art of beading alive.

Sit with your journal and work with Sense, using your feelings, understanding, common sense, awareness, brightness, sanity, and self-esteem. Write a letter to yourself about the lesson of Sense.

Example: I am a person who works with feelings. It takes a lot of understanding of myself and how I fit into the world in order for me to help others and see life as a good thing. I look deep within my common sense and use the collective thoughts of my elders and ancestors to feel and know a sense of life in its fullness. Through prayer, I have a sense of awareness of the voice of Great Spirit. My vision is my brightness that warms my heart and makes me proud of the hard work done to come to the place I am today as a woman, wife, and shaman. Through my pets and love for teaching, I have a strong sense of my sanity. With the esteem of self, and strong guidance from my mom, I smile and keep the wind to my back, living a good life.

This is the process of the lesson of Sense.

Power Medicine

Power is brought about through the lesson of Sense. There is negative Power and positive Power. Power Medicine is positive. It is night and it is dark. The darkness has one guarantee—that light shall come. It is within that Sense of light and it is within making sense and having common sense that the medicine of Power is brought into place. Why, what, when, where, and how are the only questions within Power. Power places an object in motion. It places your life on a road of movement. But you have to have common sense and apply it—taking time to make sense—in order to attain Power. When there is no Sense, there is no Power. When there is no light and only darkness, the power of dark is empty. It is dull compared to the Power of light. Lightness is sparkle. Lightness is bright. And brightness is the grandest Power of all.

Aho.

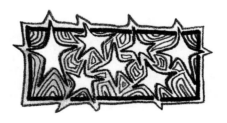

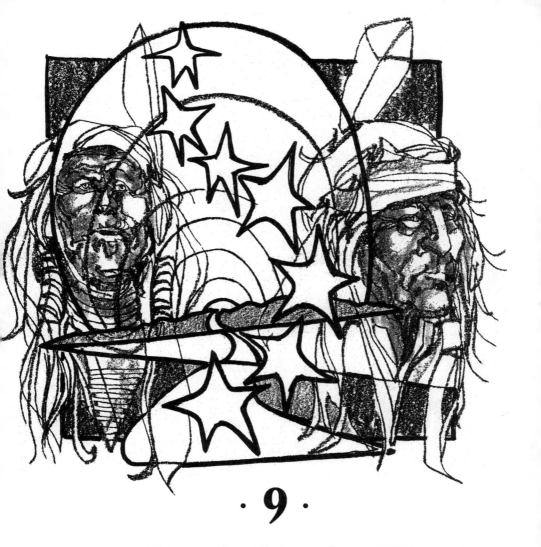

· 9 ·

THE DANCE OF THE
GREAT WATERFALL

Before me I see a medicine wheel. I see the east section with seven
medicines and seven lessons. I see the South, the emotional section, with
seven medicines and seven lessons. I see the West, with seven medicines
and seven lessons. I see the North, with seven medicines and seven lessons.
And in the center, I see the symbol of Great Spirit, the Song of seven stones
of all seven colors.

The students light candles all over the wheel. There is great joy, dancing, memories. Each student is wearing a shirt that is white and has circles with symbols, colors, beads, sequins, embroidery—much beauty has come. I breathe in and out. I feel high spirits all around me. Behind each student I see tall, slender, pale-colored spirits with enormous wings. As the students light their candles of prayer and hang their prayer ties, I have a feeling of Complete. I know that the lesson of Complete is at hand. I listen carefully and hear a soft rain. I see the colors of fall; the aspen is just turning yellow. I hear the gurgling and babbling of the water, the trickling sounds of the creek. Before me I see the walkway alongside the river. I follow it across the road and then walk along the creek as it winds its way up the hill. I pass the gate with the little sign that says *Heaven*. I remember those days. I turn and look at the old two-story house. I look behind me at the river rushing by. I follow the creek. I hear a dancing flute, weaving its sounds in the wind. I smell a fire of fresh hickory. I hear the water crashing down.

A great pleasure comes over me, a feeling of delight. I cross the creek and up ahead I see an enormous waterfall—a huge, monstrous waterfall. It rushes over the side of the cliff and falls, bursting with enthusiasm and laughter. High spirits and delight are everywhere.

I hear a familiar chant: "Aho, ahey, hey yeh, ha ha." I know that sound. I can feel that sound in my very soul. I take a deep breath and relax. Before me I see a soft mist, pale, pale colors—pinks and yellows, blues and greens. I step through the mist—through the waterfall—and stand in a familiar place of happiness. I feel great joy. There is camp; there is home. I see Grandmother and Grandfather Wolf, and they wave. Grandfather motions for me to come. I run to the side of the waterfall where he stands in all his brightness and she stands in all of her lovingness. Such good nature they have. Such fairness. I hug them and they hug me back.

"Granddaughter, we have missed you."

"Oh, Grandmother and Grandfather, I have missed you so much."

I watch Grandfather's tail sway softly back and forth. I look at the intensity in his face. He snarls, raises his lip, and then lets it drop in happiness and quietness.

"Granddaughter, I am glad you have come. It is time for me to tell you the story of the snake and the shark. It is time for you to cross through the Great Waterfall, to walk within the sacred circle of the bones."

"Grandfather, I'm not sure that I can do that. The waterfall is very scary to me. It's too big."

"Granddaughter, don't let it scare you. You know how he is," Grandmother says.

"I want you to be ready at sunset and join me down the path. Find me by the high pile of firewood, and we will talk. Go with your Grandmother now, and rest."

I follow Grandmother into the house. Camp is always such a wonderful place to be. You step into the kitchen and there are smells of jelly, of pie baking, the aroma of eucalyptus and fresh herbs drying—dill, rosemary, thyme. It is a magical place where Grandfather has stars hanging from the ceiling—stars carved out of wood, stars made out of rock, stars cascading down in all colors, where he has gathered them, carved them from stone and tied them, where he has made them from wood and painted them with blackberry and cherry juice, and rose hips. He made them for Grandmother—stars out of dried yellow flowers. The whole ceiling is lined with herbs and stars cascading down.

Grandmother taps the wooden table and says, "Sit. I'll make you a cup of tea." We drink chamomile and rose hips tea and chat. I have many things to tell her about Yellow Bird and the things I have learned in my journey through the emotions.

"Grandmother, did you know Anger? Grandmother, did you know Acceptance? Grandmother, I learned about Happy."

She just nods and says, "Yes, I know."

She has such a beautiful way of nodding, and the light reflects off her silver-white hair. Such a dignified old wolf, she is.

"Granddaughter, you will be meeting Grandfather soon. What he has to say to you is not easy. He has the Sacred Circle of the two-legged, the choice of life, for you to endure. Many two-leggeds are lost in the wind. They are broken and the fire burns away. What is inside? There are those who call to be a hollow bone and those who wish to work with prayers and be sober. The work is hard, Granddaughter—the way of your mother and father, the Great Wolf. The way of Great has come for you today. First, Grandfather will have wise words to say. I must give you something," and she hands me a bundle. It is soft, made out of buffalo skin. I feel it. It has something lumpy and bumpy inside.

"Don't open it, Granddaughter. Take it to Grandfather, and listen."

I leave the house and work my way along the trail. I look, listen, and smell as he has taught me, working my way back in through the woods, in the scrub oaks, in the cottonwood, along the creek. I listen for the snapping and crackling of fire. I see evening turn to night and up ahead of me is the big fire. I hear the drum. The night glistens. The stars speak louder than ever. I watch them drop from the sky—a red one, a cluster of green ones, a grouping of blues, some yellows and greens. I hear the enormous waterfall

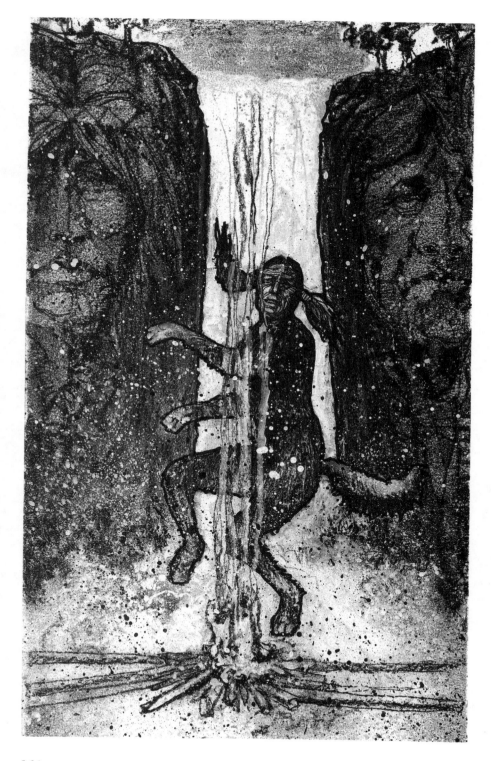

cascading over the rocks. And there is Grandfather, dancing around the fire—proud and strong—a vibrant wolf.

My mind drifts. I turn to see if Dark Eyes is anywhere near, but I don't see him. It is quiet there by the fire, with just Grandfather dancing. His intense yellow eyes see me. He lifts his lip in a snarl and a grin. I come towards him.

"Sit, Granddaughter," he says, "and listen. Listen to the night and the dance of the stars." The stars twinkle and glitter. It is great.

"I have a story to tell you," he says. "Have a stump."

I sit on the stump. The fire is very hot, and Grandfather is strong and warm as always. He sits, in all his wolfness.

"It is Great. Great is the leader; great is critical; it's serious, it's lofty. It's countless, unlimited, and spacious. All of these attributes are yours, Granddaughter. For many years, you have followed your vision of the sun, the moon, and the seven stars and you have never once asked about your parents. You have never once come to me and asked me to tell you the story of your parents and who they are."

Oh, I feel an emptiness inside me when he says that. "I didn't want to, Grandfather. I don't want to know. I've been on the Earth enough to know that it is often spoken of—the story of the evil and the story of the wolf. They always tie the wolf and evil together."

"Yes, that they do, Granddaughter. Evildoers don't want to tell the truth about the wolf, that it's a leader, that it's a teacher. They don't want anyone to know about Star Medicine."

"Who *are* they, Grandfather?"

"Conscience," he says. "Conscience, guilt, anguish, and despair. Anguish and despair once took over. They devoured conscience. And when they spat it out, they left it tainted. They left it with its ability to be *un*, to be the *un*conscience. In the underworld, the *un*conscience lives. There it is the un-limited of Great which is to be unconditional. There will be no boundaries, there will be no respect. There will be no limits and no expectations! When you overcome and understand the *un*, you are Great. You move within the depth of burgundy. The color has a solid belief and teaching—the way of the wolf—one who leads others to the path of emotional healing."

"Sometimes, Grandfather, these things of emotion are very hard for me to understand. Sometimes the stories of spirit are hard for me to understand."

"Ask me about your parents, Wolf."

"I have memories, Grandfather. I remember a cracking, a splitting; I remember flashes of light. I remember the deafening silence. I remember the cold emptiness. I don't want to ask any more."

He takes a deep breath and looks at me. He says, "You must go now, go deeper behind the waterfall. Walk a long way into the mist. You must seek out the Snake Man. You'll know him by the raven on his shoulder."

Grandfather rises and continues to move around the fire. He marches on in a dance step. He puts a foot down and says, "Lofty." He puts another one down and says, "Countless." He dances and his leg rattles click in the night.

"Leave now, Granddaughter. Behind the Great Waterfall, go deeper into the mist. Go past the purple mist, the one that lies next to burgundy, and follow the burgundy mist. Each color mist is a road. Beyond the burgundy mist you will come to the Snake Man. You will hear about the Sacred Circle of the two-legged, the choice of life. Go, Granddaughter, behind the Great Waterfall." He strikes the drum deliberately—tap, tap, tap tap. I know I have to move on.

A stick is lying on the ground before me. It has two heads, a black wolf and a white wolf. It is so familiar. I reach down and grab it, and as I do, it lifts me into the air. It spins me around and around. I am engulfed in purple mist, deep and dark. Then burgundy mist is all around me. I dance with the stick, beyond the mist, beyond the Great Waterfall.

I hear the soft sounds of the stars calling me back.

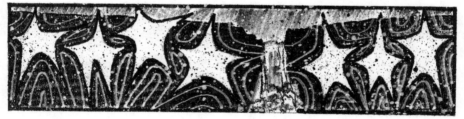

The Emotional Teachings of Joy

Make a mini-wheel and place Joy in the center. In the spirit section, place peace. In the feelings section, place happiness. In the totality section, place quiet. In the concept section, place gratification.

Joy is enjoyment, it is pleasure, it is delight, happiness, peace, quiet. It is enthusiasm, high spirits, good nature, laughter, innocence, fairness, brightness, and bold color.

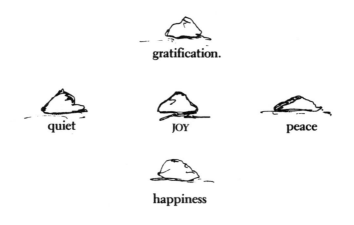

gratification.

quiet   JOY   peace

happiness

Working in the spirit section of your mini-wheel for Joy, list what is peace for you.

Example: My spirit of Joy is knowing. To me, knowing that I can walk through life and make mistakes and cause pain, because I am human—but can always start over and do better and try harder. It is within my lesson of Clarity and Sense that I have learned everything will be okay—that this new time I try I will be clearer and I can succeed. When I write, I have to make corrections, and each time I do, I become clearer. Knowing to me is blue. It is fresh and soft. I feel great comfort.

In the feelings section of Joy, list what your happiness is.

Example: Happiness to me is a quiet Sunday on the lake, fishing, sitting with a cold Coke, a good friend, and my dog. These feelings of happiness bring Joy to my life.

List the totalities of Joy, list your quietness.

Example: When I teach and see my students having a good time, answering questions, and finding peace within themselves, I am complete. I have a feeling of wholeness. When I hear them find their answers, I feel worthy to teach.

In the section of concept, list the things that gratify you.

Example: I have spent many hours and years in prayer, believing Great Spirit will open the minds of all who come to learn and achieve. I look at the twenty-some years I have taught and there is much enjoyment and enlightenment in my heart. I have a great love and respect for the growth and power felt by my students.

Work with your mini-wheel of Joy and bring yourself to a quiet enthusiasm. I advise, as always, that you use a dictionary and thesaurus to get a deeper and fuller understanding of your language. Enjoy the work with Joy!

Aho.

Ceremony of the Great Waterfall

Tools: *You'll need a garden hose close to a tree limb so you can hang the hose over it or over a rail on a porch, or you can put up a pole and wire the garden hose to it, so it can make a waterfall. You can use the shower inside your house also, but it's better to be outdoors. You'll need your spirit journal and pen, your smudge bowl, and sage.*

The Ceremony of the Great Waterfall is a ceremony of Joy. Here you can look at your inner self and the things that are real for you, that bring about your Greatness, that allow you to open up to your Joy.

1. In your spirit journal, answer the question "What brings you Joy?" List all the things that bring joy to you. That would be things that give you pleasure or delight, peace, quietness, enthusiasm, laughter. List the things that give you Joy.
   The second part of this question is "What makes you happy?" These are actions that please you, that satisfy you, that delight you, that are positive— things that are fruitful. Look within your life and list what makes you happy.

2. Now list what takes it away. What takes your Joy away? What makes you unhappy?

3. Describe your being in high spirits, what makes you feel full and understand what richness is.

   Example: *Taking a long walk with my wolf, watching the deer run in the* *early morning. That gives me the kind of fulfillment that opens a burst of energy in me. It gives me the creative energy to write.*

4. Describe your good nature.

Example: *I'm walking in the park one day with my dog, and my dog is being admired. The person approaches me and says, "I can't help but notice your dog playing Frisbee, and I wish I had one like him." I can't give my dog to the person, because I can't be separated from my dog, but I do allow the person to play with the dog.*

5. **The ceremony.** Turn the water on and start your waterfall. Let the garden hose become the source of the waterfall. Watch the water bounce and burst open for you, giving you the opportunity to step into Great. Look at the Greatness of the cleansing of the water. Watch it hit and pound on the ground. Watch it rush out of the hose or the showerhead. Stand under it and feel your Greatness. Allow the water, the Great Waterfall, to wash away everything that takes away your happiness and joy. Let any thoughts of negativity and self-belittlement fall with the water.

While you are under the water, breathe in—breathe in the unlimited. Walk hand in hand with Great. Hold in your mind that Great is spacious and allow spacious to be your personality. See yourself as countless and vast. Visualize yourself as important. Hold yourself as main and lofty. Listen to the water running and know and live with joy in your heart.

Spirit Shirt Vision of the Snake

Go someplace where it is quiet and you won't be disturbed. Sit or lie down, and close your eyes. Have your spirit journal ready. Breathe in and out, and relax. You'll hear a hissing and the rattle of a rattlesnake. Listen to the hissing sound and breathe and relax. Listen to the rattling sound. In front of you, you'll see a waterfall, an enormous waterfall, with water billowing over the cliff, crashing down, hitting the rocks and splashing. Feel the ground shaking from the waterfall. As you look at the waterfall, you'll see your symbol. Remember what it looks like. Bring it back and draw a green circle with a burgundy circle inside it, and in the center of that put your symbol. You're ready to paint it on your shirt now.

Your spirit shirt is complete at this point, with your seven symbols. It is ready for you to sew on bits of ribbon and to embroider it, bead it, put sequins on it, or paint other things on it along with your symbols. Your spirit shirt is ready to celebrate and to wear in honor of your spirit knowledge of the South through your emotions, getting a better understanding of your emotions and looking at the depth of your Strength, your Success, your Vision, your Beauty, your Healing, your Power, and your Greatness. This finishes the visions within Star Medicine for your spirit shirt.

Aho.

Completed Spirit Shirt with Symbols

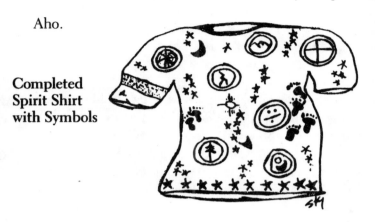

Dance Stick

Tools: *A stick; a carving, whittling, or pocket knife; paints in red, orange, yellow, green, blue, purple, and burgundy; plus a black marker.*

There are many kinds of dance sticks. They are connected with your inner animal spirit. Your animal could be an eagle and your dance stick could take on that form, as does the one in the picture, with an eagle's talon, claw, or foot at the end of it, which could be carved or painted on the stick. The stick could be in the shape of a horse or a horse's head, or like the one described in the story—with two heads of different animals.

1. Sit quietly with the stick that you have chosen, and feel the spirit of your inner animal. You'll see it in your mind—four times it will come to you. Each time you see the animal, remember it, and when you have seen it four times, you'll know it to be the spirit of your dance stick. You could have—instead of an eagle or horse—a dance stick that is an elk, a turtle, a hawk, a dragonfly, a frog, an owl, or a snake. These are all animals that are connected to your medicines. You could also have other animals—winged ones and crawlies—that are connected to your lessons, such as a hummingbird, an otter, a butterfly, a slug, a weasel, a whale, or a shark. When you feel that you have your spirit animal, go on.

2. Look at the four movements of your stick. The first movement of your stick is unlimited. Write in your spirit journal what unlimited means to you and connect it to your spirit animal.

> *Example: The elk that I dance with in my spirit stick is totally unlimited. It makes no demands, has no expectations, and has no rules that it places on me and none that I place on it. Therefore, I can feel the fullness of its spirit.*

The second movement is important. Write down what important is to you and connect it to your dance stick.

> *Example: I have made a dance stick out of a turtle. The turtle is very important to me, for it represents the Earth. It represents all the teachings of the star system that are connected to the Earth Mother. To me, the importance of carrying the turtle keeps me connected and grounded, for groundedness is a medicine of the turtle.*

List the things that are important to you about your spirit that you have in your dance stick.

Third, list what is serious to you, connected to the animal, and to your dance stick.

Dance Stick

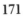

Example: The hawk is very serious to me, because it is a connection to the Osage people, for the hawk is a symbol within the Osage. I would dance with the hawk in a serious way, for it is my family.

Fourth, list what is Lofty about the stick. Describe what is lofty to you and connect it to the stick.

Example: The owl is very lofty. It is revered and feared by many. It would be great, high, and lofty for me to carry the owl, for I would carry with me secrets. I would have the ability to be invisible and walk in the dark without being seen as the light spirit that I am.

List the lofty things that go along with your dance stick.

3. Carve your dance stick, paint it, draw on it. Decorate it, place skin on it from the animal you worked with, or fur or feathers, or objects such as mirrors and bells. Mirrors project back evil, the negative. They reflect away things that you don't wish to have in your life. Bells give you a protection, quietness. Bring forth your dance stick.

4. Using a dance stick. You can use it when you choose to dance a ceremonial dance. You can hang it on the wall and have it there to dance with in your mind. A dance stick is an object of power, a spirit stick that helps you to understand the dances of your emotions. It is given to you to respect and to honor.

Aho.

The Process of the Lesson of Complete

Within the process of the Lesson of Complete you are working with whole, solid, intact, real, essential, total, entire, unbroken, sound, and full. To understand Complete, work with the vision of the Great Waterfall.

1. In your mind recall the water running from the waterfall, or the water hose that you stood under physically. Know that it is a place where you can wash away your negative thoughts and feelings. In your spirit journal list your weaknesses. List what you think is broken in yourself. List what seems

empty, what seems incomplete, what is stupid and silly, what is limited and unhappy.

2. Explain how you can bring about change in each of these negatives, why you would want to change them, why you would want to let go of your incompletion, your silly and stupid. Explain why you would want to wash yourself clean and clear.

3. As before, but in spirit now, step under the waterfall and let go. Let these inadequacies—this weakness and brokenness, incompletion and emptiness, silliness, stupidity, and unhappiness—all be washed away, so that you are clean and clear.

4. See yourself being coated in water. As the water comes down, it will be a color. Bring down red for wholeness. Bring down green for solidity. Bring down blue for being intact. Bring down white for being real. Feel yourself becoming happy and remember what you wrote happiness to be for yourself. See yourself as unlimited. Allow your spirit to dance with your stick. See yourself as sincere and solid. You have brought about the process of the lesson of Complete.

5. The final step is to see yourself sitting in the medicine wheel, very sacred, very quiet, very much in the emotion of Acceptance, straight and full.

Great Medicine

Great medicine is that of Complete. One of the greatest things that happens in your life is to Complete—to be Complete, to have, to know, to have Complete, to be, to do, to bring about Complete. Complete is the movement of Great. Great medicine is the opportunity, once again, to have Complete. It is your ability to have Clarity and utilize the Disciplines of life that come from your Vision, and open up the opportunities that are your Success. Great is a movement of Strength. It is Beauty in its fullness, which brings about totality within Power. It is understanding that, with Joy, Great is in its fullness.

Aho.

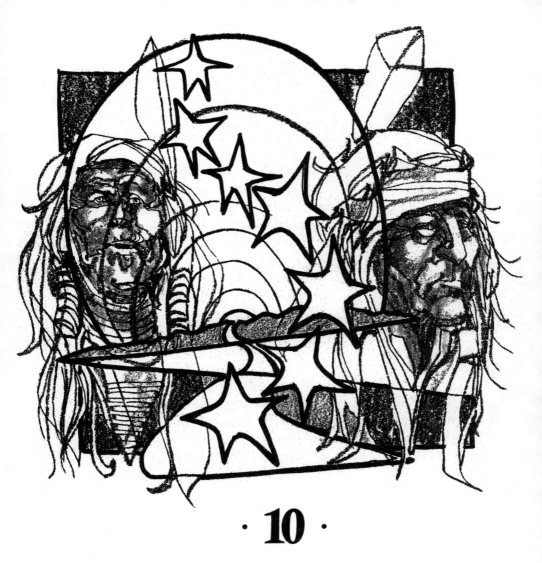

· 10 ·

THE SACRED CIRCLE OF THE TWO-LEGGED CHOICE OF LIFE

Before me I see a familiar path. It is almost hidden in a very dark burgundy mist. Then moonlight pierces the mist and I see the burgundy color. The mist lifts and becomes pale mauve. In front of me I see a medicine wheel. I see the candles glowing in the night. I see each stone—stars light the tops of them. There are red stones, orange ones, purple ones, green ones, and in the center I see the buffalo skull. I see the smudge bowl in the center, with smoke circling in the air, spiraling, and I smell sweet grass and sage. On the cords around the medicine wheel I see prayer ties draped, hanging over the lines. I feel the sacredness of this place.

Outside the circle I see a blackness—it is pitch-black. I hear the chanting of an old one, a voice in the night. Around the medicine wheel the students dance. I say to them, "It is your choice now." I hear the eagle-bone whistle. I hear the calling of the spirit. I look around on both sides to see what elder has emerged. There is no one, just the roll of thunder, the quiet of the night. Darkness.

"Each of you has come and you have entered through the east gate, spun around and lifted your hands to Great Spirit, Grandmother, Grandfather, and asked if they understood your prayers. Have you gone to the Great Waterfall? Have you stepped into the Grandness of Great and looked at how simple Greatness is? Have you let go of your false pride?" The students stare at me, questions in their eyes.

We prepare to dance around the medicine wheel, to celebrate their Dance of the Rainbow Self. They are wearing their spirit shirts and the symbols are known in their hearts. To the West my brother wolf is playing his flute, his head dropped down, his black hat covering his face. He plays a song into the night—"Two Flutes" it is called. He plays the parts of the two flutes. It is sacred here tonight in the dark. There are tiny twinkles, the song of the stars.

The students dance around the wheel in Joy, holding their spirit sticks in the air, carrying their dance sticks and holding on to their Power, reaching for the stars to heal their scars. I hear the call of the Raven. I walk over the wheel, stepping out above it. I step high into the sky and walk on the stars into the spirit world.

"I hear you! Wait, Raven! I hear you!"

The Raven flies on and I follow. I am standing in the dark of burgundy and there, in front of me, I see an old one. Long, gray braids. Black hat putted down. Ribbon shirt, blue jeans, and boots. On his shoulder sits the Raven.

"You must be the one. You must be the one that Grandfather spoke of. I must speak to you. You will tell me of the Sacred Circle of the Two-Legged?"

"Hmmm," he says. He sits in a circle of cornmeal. In the center is a very

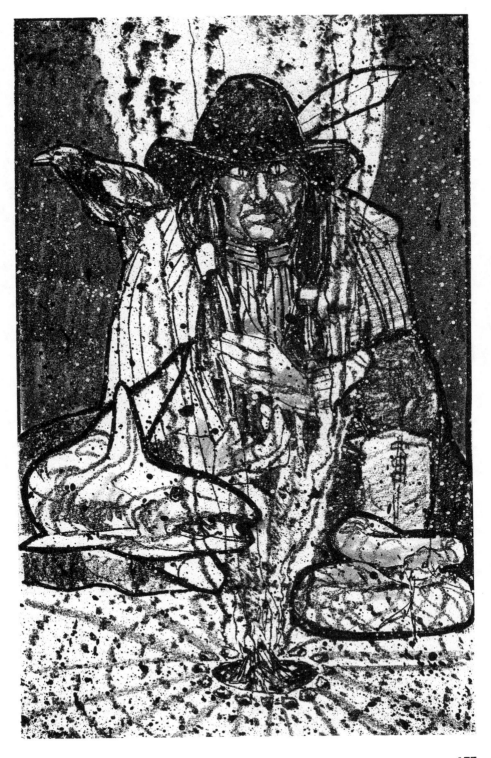

tiny fire pit, with a little bitty fire, intricately made of tiny twigs. Small stones of turquoise circle the edges of the fire. "Yes, I have something to say."

His face is long and narrow, very Native. He lifts it, and the fire reflects in his face. I look into his eyes.

"I must tell you the story of the snake and the shark, the ripping and tearing of Complete, as it burns away all your negatives. It is a lesson that your Grandfather chose for me to tell you. I must tell you the story of the snake."

As he says this, the fire pops and grows brighter. I see his eyes—they are the eyes of a snake. He drops his head and shadows fall over his face. The Raven flies off.

"The lesson of Complete is never fulfilled until you have walked on the Earth as a two-legged. Each one of us must be a bone."

Behind him is a large, billowing shadow—huge. At first I think it is a man. Now I can see it is a grizzly. Maybe it is just a black bear—no, it's a brown bear. It is a grizzly. It stands behind him and raises its paws up high above him. It has long nails. It shows its teeth and looks me in the eye. I feel a coldness behind me. I hear the black horse. I turn, and there is Death. I look the other way, and there is the White Owl Woman. In front of me is the old man; behind him the grizzly is snarling in my face.

"Don't worry, Wolf. It's simply the West," the old man says. "You have walked into the shimmering yellow of the aspen; it is time for the fall. That's why we have this soft rain. It is my part of the wheel, now. I open the door within the Sacred Circles, the study of the two-legged. "Do you know the story of the snake and the shark?"

"No. The answer is no," I say. "Much like I don't know you."

"Oh, excuse me." His voice is gruff and aged. "My name is Snake Man. I have come to guide you to the doorway, for within the Sacred Circles is the Grandness. When you step through the Waterfall, you step into the realm of knowing in spirit. You face the Rainbow Warrior, the guardian of the realm of knowing in spirit, and are given a gift. The Rainbow Warrior comes to give you rebirth within your spirit life."

I have stepped into Clarity.

"It doesn't matter who our physical family is," I tell him. "It doesn't matter if we have identity, heritage, or tradition. What matters is Clarity, and I know the lesson of Discipline. When we know those two lessons, we stand in completeness, Snake Man."

He points at the shark and says, "Complete. Life and death. The Great White Shark. Two of the most evil—the snake and the shark. Yes," he smiles. "Look at the pain. Well, you'll see, with the teaching of the bones. Your life is all in the name of what is limited, as your body tells the story. You must walk within the west gate—in the medicine wheel, which is guarded by the Bear."

He snaps his fingers and the sun is setting. One minute dark, and now sunset!

"The truth of the snake and the shark is simple. They are human reality. They are within Great and Complete. Matters of life and death. The snake and the shark are often seen as evil ones, when we are actually teachers. We protect the Earth by being quick and full of knowing," Snake Man says.

"Grandfather Wolf sent me here to hear something you know, but I feel you are talking in riddles," I say.

"Well, Wolf, do you know the Sacred Circles of life?"

My head begins to spin. I see the red eyes of the shark. I hear chanting and bells rattling. I drift off to sleep as Snake Man talks on. I awaken to a raven looking me in the face. It flies from the East to the West. Standing there before me is a huge bear. I hear words from behind me, Snake Man's voice.

"You, Wolf, teach about life, death, grief, evil—live in two worlds, spirit and physical. Face your parents, Wolf."

My mind is still spinning. I feel myself floating off into a dark blue mist. I can hear the clicking and the rattling of bones. Before me I see my two worlds—a world of spirit, dancing stars, and singing wind—and a world of teaching, students, the dance of the Rainbow Self, emotions, Acceptance, Disgust, Sad, Happy, Anger, Fear, and Joy.

Seven two-leggeds sit in a circle, one with tears, one with laughter, one looking for a vision, one on a journey. I look around and see the Snake's eyes. They are warm and kind.

"You look tired, Wolf," he says. "You try hard. Soon you will be meeting the Bear. He is the brother of the Eagle, the brother of the Wolf, the brother of the Coyote. Soon you will receive the teachings of the hollow bone. There are great mysteries in life, and the greatest mystery of all is that of the bone."

Beside Snake Man is an old woman with a blanket around her. It is pulled up around her head. She has a very ancient, wrinkled face, a very solid face, with small beady black eyes, no teeth. She stands quiet and soft by his side.

"Do I know you?" I ask.

She just looks at me, no words.

"Does she know about evil? Will she teach me?" I ask.

"Evil? No," says Snake Man. "She is about the circle of the sacred ones. Remember your parents . . ."

"I remember my parents. I remember them just fine," I say. "I remember the things I don't want to know, because if I bring these things into my emotions I have choice. There will be physical or spiritual. Since I'm here with you in the spirit and everything is peace, then why should I want to become physical and leave the spirit world?"

Smoke floats around Snake Man and he is gone in a mist of color. Green and orange, blue, and white spin around me. I hear a soft voice, the voice of the old woman.

"I am Rock, old woman Rock, nature, choice, ceremony, change, and proof—real and grand. And these are the teachings of the Sacred Circles. "Follow me, find me," the voice drifts off.

I see the mist of the Great Waterfall in front of me. I step through and sit on a large rock there by the water.

"My parents, they are emotions, Grandfather Wolf. They are life and death. But are they evil?" I call out for Grandfather Wolf. "Are you here? Are my parents evil?"

Grandfather Wolf steps out of the mist. "Oh, Wolf, you are the path of life and death. All is within the dance of the Rainbow Self. You are the sun, moon, and the seven stars. No, they're not evil," he says with a smile. "I sent you to see Snake Man, for he knows how to change. I want you to change your doubt. You should never have any doubt in life. Doubt is an open window. It allows anger to come in. Doubt is a change point. Do you understand, Wolf? You need change as a medicine."

"So my whole experience with anger is my choice?" I ask.

"You have always had a choice. You have two worlds to live with—to walk the walk as a two-legged with your gifts and follow your vision—or to doubt . . ."

Grandfather looks at me with an ornery grin, eyes sparkling. He says, "You know, if you leave a window open, a vampire might come to dinner."

"Grandfather, I'm not afraid of vampires."

His laughter fills my heart with warmth.

"Grandfather," I say, "this experience of Great—this opportunity to stand with the Great Waterfall—I just want you to know I look forward to choice and change."

Suddenly a whirlwind comes up and I can't hear him speak. The dust spins in colors and he disappears.

I hear the soft sounds of the stars calling me back.

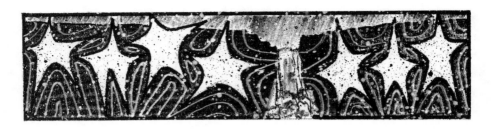

The Vision of the Physical Self

1. Ancestors and others. List in your journal how you see your ancestors. Describe them very carefully. List your elders—your mom, your dad, brothers, sisters, aunts and uncles, grandparents, cousins, anyone else important in your family life. Give a solid description of what they are to you, what they are like, and what they gave you—your physical self.

2. Describe our species. Describe "human." List and describe everything you can about yourself as a human.

> *Example: Are you African-American, are you Native American; are you Jewish; are you white? List your height—are you tall, are you short, are you fat, are you skinny?*

3. List your clan. Are you from the bears? Are you from the wolves, are you from the horses, are you from the cats? If you don't know your clan, look at what you identify with and claim that as your clan.

4. What is your element? Are you air? Are you fire? Water? Or are you earth? If you do not know that, then sit quietly and know which you are drawn to. It is easier and faster to go within yourself to find out which it is than to try to connect it to astrology or any other system. Just know your element and who you are.

> *Example: I am from the water. My secondary is air.*

How do you feel about the air and the water, the earth and the fire? List the different and varied feelings you have and you will understand yourself better. The depth of your physical being becomes clear as you examine air, fire, earth, and water.

5. Your sexual identity. Is it male or female? Explain why you feel you are a male or a female. Get past the physicality, the things on your body that make you a male or female, and explain the reality and your acceptance of it. Ask yourself whether you are you what you want? What is the strength of your sexual identity? Would you change it? What is the energy of your sexuality? Look at your physicality.

6. Identify yourself physically.

> *Example: My ancestors are of the stars and my elders are Native American, English, Osage, and Cherokee. My species is human. It is large and strong. My clan is that of the wolf.*

The Process of Bone Medicine

Tools: *Four bones; cornmeal; smudge bowl; cedar; sage; journal and pen.*

You'll need various bones. To do the process correctly, you'll need a bone that represents life, one that represents death, one that represents human, and one that represents spirit.

Build a cornmeal circle, smudge the area with the smoke of cedar and sage, and place the bones inside.

Take your journal and describe the bone of life. What are the limits of life? Journal your feelings about death. How do you understand death? List your feelings about the bone that represents human. List your feelings about the bone that represents spirit.

> *Example: Bone is life. It is a Sacred Circle of life—from dust comes life, from life comes death, and so it goes. As death comes, we are returned to dust and life comes from the Earth. The Sacred Circle of life begins with death. We the two-legged are born to life from death as a bone, which is our life as a human. Our bone is the sacred walk of the spirit, which finds its truth within the hollow bone we know as life. As we walk, each of us has the chance to be a hollow bone and to allow Great Spirit to speak through us.*

The Vision of the Sacred Bone

You'll need a quiet place where you can sit and not be disturbed. Breathe in and out, and close your eyes. Before you you'll see a gateway to the East with a red flag on the top. Step up to it, hold your hands in the air and spin in through the gate. Spinning clockwise, you'll step into the wheel. There in front of you you'll see the buffalo skull, forming the center. You'll see the circle of stones spiraling around the center—red, orange, yellow, green, blue, purple and burgundy. Move clockwise. Standing at the South, honor the gate by raising your hands. Give thanks for the South and step past each Medicine Stone, honoring your Strength, your Success, your Vision. Hold dear in your heart your Beauty, your Healing, your Power, and your Greatness.

Turn, look to the center and, seeing the line going to the South, you'll know that your lessons in the emotions are strong. Give thanks for your emotions—Acceptance, Disgust, Happy and Sad, Anger, Fear and Joy.

Walk clockwise to the right and there you'll see another gateway. It will have a blue flag on it. Raise your hands in the air to honor it. Listen quietly for the spirit of the West. Look for the Bear, listen for his message. Hear the voice of the West. You'll hear the song of the stars quietly and softly calling you back.

Take out your journal and in it describe what spirit means to you. Write about the soft song of the stars that calls you. Write all your feelings. If you need help, go to your mini-wheels and look at the feelings sections. Look at the different feelings within each mini-wheel.

List your totalities from the mini-wheels. List the concept you have from your mini-wheel of your physicality, of your sacred bone, of your physical self.

Allow yourself to dance—always to dance—the Dance of the Rainbow Self. Lift your dance stick high in the air. Count coup on your fears and dance them.

Aho.

Medicine Voices

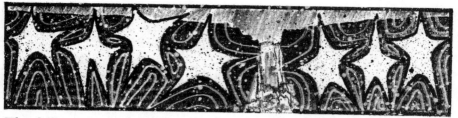

The following interpretations are mine. They may help you understand your vision and the depth of your walk as a two-legged.

Medicine Words

Strength—Red. Strength is stamina, comprehension, and solidity in what you do. It is your ability, your standing—taking each thing that comes your way and being able to handle it with Confidence, knowing that you've done your best. Strength is holding within you the red flame that glows in the night, setting your jaw solid and standing with honor.

Success—Orange. Success in men or women is measured by their family. It is measured by the good words others say. Success is never what you say, but how you walk. It is being able to say, "I did the best I can do and there is nothing else I can do." Wealth and prosperity within Success are your family. Success is also achievement. It is solidity, your Balance.

Vision—Yellow. Vision is a gift of Great Spirit. It is bestowed on you as a pathway, as guidance, as an opportunity to look into the future with a picture. Vision could be a blackboard with a drawing of a tree, a mountain, and a river, and that may be all you'll need to guide you. Vision is a ceremony. It is a haunting. It is a spirit calling your name. You look and there it is. You ask of it, "What are you?" And it gives back an answer.

Beauty—Green. Beauty is as beauty does. As you do, so are you beautiful. As another sees you and breathes you in and holds you for the breath that you are, that is Beauty.

Healing—Blue. Healing is knowing. Healing is drawing from inside your truth, changing, curing, transforming. The grandest of all healings is to transform from illness to truth.

Power—Purple. It is not a trip—not holding and lording it over others. Power is letting go of your false pride and being humble. Power is looking within yourself and using that humility as a strength for building a ladder that carries you into the sky, where you can walk on the stars. Power is having the ability to stand beyond abuse and neglect, judgment, reprimands, racism, and be yourself. To exist and remain to become an elder is Power.

Great—Burgundy. Great is the massive amount that comes down on your head every day, which you endure—known as your existence. No matter how bad the news is, or how badly people speak of you, you are still yourself. Great is the Sacred Circle, the Sacred Hoop, the hollow bone that you can be yourself. Great is your name. Great is your moment.

Colors

Red. Confidence, Strength, Nurture, Color, Absolute, Illumination, Beginning, Accountability.

Orange. Balance, Success, Energy, Choice, Correct, Following, Proceeding, Responsibility.

Yellow. Creativity, Vision, Ceremony, Prayer, Ideal, Solidity, Sincerity.

Green. Growth, Beauty, Change, Quiet, Perfect, Faith, Innocence, Honest.

Blue. Truth, Healing, Proof, Tranquility, Clarity, Introspection, Depth, Faithful, Understanding.

Purple. Wisdom, Power, Real, Knowledge, Pure, Commitment.

Burgundy. Impeccable, Great, Grand, Mystery, Will, The Path.

White. Silver, Spiritual, All.

Black. Gold, Totality, Wholeness, Physical, Monetary, Mass, Material.

Lesson Words

Clarity—Red. Clarity is a doorway. It is crystal; it is known; it is opening to reality. It gives you your uniqueness. Clarity is translucent, luminous, clean, and honest. Clarity does not make a thing bigger or smaller; it's not for building or shrinking. It shows it like it is.

Poise—Orange. Poise is dignity. It is a right, which each of us is given by Great Spirit, Grandmother, Grandfather—a right to breathe, to struggle, to survive. Poise is standing evenly matched in Balance—right there—knowing your point.

Discipline—Yellow. The lesson of Discipline is what you heap on yourself. Pile the books higher on your head, pile the homework deeper, and reach for the top. Discipline is the reaching, the pulling from within, placing it outside, and moving. Discipline is not caving in, but standing straight.

Account—Green. Account is that cold water that hits you in the face in the morning. It is the growth of the self. Look at where you are in the wheel.

Fact—Blue. Fact is the knowing—belief and understanding. You learn from experience and experience is Fact.

Sense—Purple. You can look at it in many ways. You think, does it make sense? And you'll miss it. Sense is also touch. It touched you, you touched it. Sense is simple, common sense. Or you think there is one and there are truly two.

Complete—Burgundy. Complete is a Grand word. Complete is when you reach out into spirit and live in the hollowness of the bone, where you understand that spirit flows through all things. If you can't grasp that, you need to study constantly until finally you come to Complete. No one ever has the answer for you, but you do. So what is in your heart—what is so for you—is what is Complete. There are other ways to Complete—completing other people, completing what they want done. But the real Complete is yours, what flows through the hollowness.

Medicine Helpers

The following creatures are the Medicine Helpers—the four-legged, the winged ones, the hoppers, the crawlies, the swimmers. These are the spirit guides for the south section of the Rainbow Medicine Wheel.

Animal Spirit Guides

Butterfly. Beauty, circle of life, transformation.

Coyote. Playfulness, one who understands, fun, trickster, one who walks in balance, growth, youthfulness, South.

Dragonfly. Doorway, vision, knowing.

Elk. Strength, romance, love medicine.

Frog. Clear away, clear, a new day, joy.

Hawk. Listener, one who hears Great Spirit clearly, messenger.

Hummingbird. Happy, joy, gift.

Land Turtle. Mother, giver of life, storyteller, rainbow-maker.

Otter. Poise, walking your walk, the feminine.

Owl. Listener, one who understands, power, gift, death.

Shark. To cut through, to believe, sharp, challenge.

Slug. Steadfast, stable, sparkle, slow, steady, perseverance.

Snake. To shed, to let go of, to turn from, protector.

Weasel. Challenge, trickster, teacher.

Whale. Breath, knowing, to open.

Medicine Rocks

Agate. Courage, support, appreciation, grounding, solidity.

Amber. Memory connection, crystal, clear, clean, organizes thoughts, generates.

Amethyst. Modify, knowing, wisdom.

Flint. Protection of spirit.

Garnets. Grounding, solidity.

Gold. Attracting energy.

Obsidian. Psychic development.

Raw Rubies. Spiritual protection.

Silver. Attracting spirit.

Herbs

Cedar. Centers fear and anger, connects to Great Spirit.

Cornmeal. Sets sacred space, balances energy fields with positive energy, feeds spirit guides and spirit helpers, welcomes spirits of the light kind.

Juniper. Moves negative energy, protection.

Piñon. Protects, cleans negative energy, welcomes spirit.

Sage. Honors, cleanses, freshens, balances spirit, clears.

Sandalwood. Opens psychic ability, allows you to seek harmony.

Sweet grass. Balances, energizes, clears, reduces anxiety, centers.

Acknowledgments

I would like to acknowledge the dancers who give of themselves to put their steps forth as a language of prayer. I acknowledge all the dancers, all over the world, who dance in indigenous ways and hold true to the sacred teachings that they receive from their elders—grandmothers, grandfathers, aunties, and uncles. I can see emotions in movement and I am always grateful that you dance.

I would like to give a special acknowledgment to a very dear lady, Auntie Sue. One who holds her beliefs dear in her heart, she carries them through her sobriety, through her walk, through her memories of her father, a grass dancer—and she brings those memories back to her children and gives them to her grandchildren. I acknowledge her with all my heart.

I have a special acknowledgment to one who walks as a student, who has carried her faith and her people silent in her heart. When she walked toward me, she walked with a question, "Can you have white blood and still be Native?" I acknowledge the fact that she has danced her Star Medicine and has understood that when you reach for the stars you heal the scars. I acknowledge all of us who seek out our heritage to find the mysticism or the spirit or the understanding that allow us to feel full, to feel whole, and to ride the wind and dance among the stars.

A special thanks to Sheila Anne Barry again, for her assistance and her belief. Much love and appreciation to Joanne, Granny Jo, Dancing Spirit, for her work in helping me bring the words forth. As always, it would not happen without her magic fingers.

And acknowledgment and, as always, a great gratitude for my half side, Raven, who walks with me in fullness, in wholeness, in his totality.

To contact the Author:

Wolf Moondance
453 East Wonderview Avenue
P.O. Box 6000
Estes Park, CO 80517

Index

190